THE
OF
DIFFICULTIES

A Translation
of the *Nan Jing*

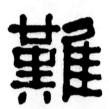

Translated
by Bob Flaws

Blue Poppy Press • Boulder, CO

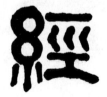

一难曰: 十二径皆有动脉, 独取寸口

Published by:
BLUE POPPY PRESS
A Division of Blue Poppy Enterprises, Inc.
5441 Western Ave., Suite 2
BOULDER, CO 80301

First Edition, March, 1999
Second Edition, March 2003
Third Edition, August 2003
Fourth Edition, November 2003
Fourth Edition, November 2004

ISBN 1-891845-07-1
LC# 98-74994

COMP Designation: Denotative translation

Printed at C&M Press, Denver, CO
10 9 8 7 6 5

Preface

This book is a translation of the *Huang Di Ba Shi Yi Nan Jing (The Yellow Emperor's Eighty-one Difficulties Classic)* more commonly known simply as the *Nan Jing* or *Classic of Difficulties*. This is a collection of eighty-one questions and answers seeking to clarify difficult passages or concepts within the *Huang Di Nei Jing (The Yellow Emperor's Inner Classic)*. Chinese medical scholars believe this book was written or compiled some time in the late Han dynasty during the first or second centuries CE. Traditionally, the authorship of the *Nan Jing* is attributed to Bian Que, the legendary first acupuncturist of antiquity. However, this is historically impossible and is simply a pious fiction.

This book is important to the history and development of Chinese medicine and especially acupuncture for three reasons. First, it presents a relatively coherent system of pulse diagnosis centering on the three positions and various levels of the *cun kou* or inch mouth found on the radial artery at the styloid processes of the wrists. While there are references to a number of different systems of pulse examination mentioned in the *Nei Jing* or *Inner Classic*, none of these are sufficiently explained to be put into clinical practice with any confidence. It was the *Nan Jing* which focused Chinese doctors' attention on the inch mouth pulse and described a coherent system of examination and correspondence which is still used in several Asian and European countries to this day.

Secondly, this book presents and clarifies the clinical application of five phase theory. Five phase theory is a further evolution of yin yang theory whereby everything in the phenomenal universe corresponds to one or some combination of five basic phases. Because these five phases reminded early Westerners of the four elements of Western scholastic medicine, they were first erroneously named the five elements. However, these five are not static entities or elements but rather five stages in the evolution of any phenomenally existing thing which also engender and restrain each other in a constantly changing and dynamic way. Although Chinese Daoists and Confucianists still argue to this day over whether five phase theory and the medicine of systematic correspondences it gave rise to is a Daoist or Confucian creation, it is this system of systematic correspondence which forms the basis of almost all the other theories and practices of Chinese medicine.

And third, it is the *Nan Jing* which codifies the use of the so-called transport points existing between the elbows and fingertips and knees and toes. Sometimes referred to in English as the "antique points" or the "command points," this is a set of 60 pre-eminently important points in the practice of acupuncture. As the text explains, each of the 12 channels has a set of five points corresponding to the five phases. Since each of the five phases corresponds to one or more of the viscera and bowels, channels and vessels, directions, seasons, colors, flavors, odors, sounds, fluids, tissues, emotions, etc., and since each channel has a point corresponding to each of the five phases, by variously supplementing and draining different combinations of these five phase points, one can re-establish the dynamic balance of these five phases within the human body and between the human body and the macrocosm outside.

Therefore, the *Nan Jing* is a seminally important classic for anyone who A) is interested in Chinese pulse diagnosis, B) anyone interested in the Chinese medicine of systematic corre-spondences in general and five phase theory in particular, and C) anyone interested in Chinese acupuncture in particular. Although this book does not describe the use of Chinese medicinals, its theory of diagnosis and treatment was applied to internal medicine in the Jin-Yuan dynasties. Hence the *Nan Jing* has had a far-reaching and long-lasting impact on Chinese medicine in every country to which this medicine has traveled. In particular, the *Nan Jing* has had a huge impact on so-called Japanese Meridian acupuncture and, through the Japanese connection with Taiwan, on a number of European and American styles of acupuncture. Thus I believe that every prac-titioner of Chinese medicine and acupuncture should be familiar with this seminal classic.

Each of the questions and answers contained in this book only comprise a paragraph or two. This book is extremely pithy and succinct even by ancient Chinese standards. In old China, this classic was meant to be memorized and not just read. The style in which it was written was chosen, in part, to help such memorization. Therefore, I have tried to retain the succinctness of the original text as far as possible. Where I have had to add words other than prepositions and conjunctions not in the original text, I have done so in brackets. When I have deemed that even further explanation is necessary in order to make any sense of a word, sentence, or passage, I have added a footnote as commentary. Many line by line commentaries of the *Nan Jing* exist in Chinese. A number of these have been included in Paul U. Unschuld's scholarly translation of this text: *Medicine in China: Nan-ching, The Classic of Difficult Issues*, University of California Press, Berkeley, 1986, and I refer readers to that excellent source for further elaboration of this text.

That being said, Dr. Unschuld is not a professional practitioner of Chinese medicine or acupuncture, and many Western practitioners have long complained that his choice of words makes his translation of this important classic clinically hard to use. For instance, Unschuld translates qi as influences and the viscera and bowels as depots and palaces. I also do not think Dr. Unschuld, as a non-native English speaker, has always chosen the most direct or best English translations. His translation is much more verbose than mine. Further, I think Dr. Unschuld has made too many bracketed additions to the text, thus imposing certain interpretations on the text. Classical Chinese is inherently ambiguous, and when we render such texts too particularly, we often lose the multiple layers of meaning the author meant to suggest. If one reads the various commentaries included in Dr. Unschuld's book, one can see that the meaning and clinical implications of almost every line in this classic have been hotly debated.

As far as possible, I have used Nigel Wiseman's translational terminology as it appears in *English-Chinese Chinese-English Dictionary of Chinese Medicine*, Hunan Science & Technology

Press, Changsha, 1995. Where I disagree with one of Dr. Wiseman's word choices, I have marked and explained my divergence in a footnote. Whenever the text discusses a named acupuncture point, I first give Wiseman's suggested English translation of the name. This is then followed by the romanized spelling of the name in Pinyin and a channel and number identification, both in parentheses. These channel and number identifications are based on the World Health Organization's suggested standard acupuncture point nomenclature with the following exceptions: Lu stands for lungs; St stands for stomach; Sp stands for spleen; Ht stands for heart; Bl stands for bladder; Ki stands for kidneys; Per stands for pericardium; TB stands for triple burner; Liv stands for liver, CV stands for conception vessel; and GV stands for governing vessel.

The source texts for this translation were Unschuld's aforementioned book, which includes the Chinese text in full, the *Nan Jing* published by the Science & Technology Publishing Co., Beijing, 1996, and Xu Da-chun's *Nan Jing Jing Shi (An Elucidation of the Classic of*

Difficulties) published by the Jiangsu Science & Technology Publishing Co., 1985.

I am especially happy that Blue Poppy Press is bringing this translation out in a true pocket-book size, making it both affordable for students and easily portable for repeated study and reference. The *Nan Jing* is one of the four basic foundation texts of Chinese medicine, the other three being the *Nei Jing*, the *Shang Han Lun (Treatise on Damage [Due to] Cold)*, and the *Shen Nong Ben Cao (The Divine Farmer's Materia Medica)*. Hopefully this edition of this seminal classic will prod more Western acupuncture schools to include its study in their basic, entry-level, core curriculum.

Bob Flaws
Mach 10, 1999

Synopsis

Difficulties 1-22 deal with pulse examination.

Difficulties 23-29 deal with the channels and network vessels.

Difficulties 30-47 deal with anatomy and physiology.

Difficulties 48-61 deal with disease causes, disease mechanisms, and diagnosis.

Difficulties 62-68 deal with the 60 transport points.

Difficulties 69-81 deal with supplementing and draining with needles.

One

Difficulty One says: Within the 12 channels, all have stirring vessels.[1] [Yet] one chooses only the *cun kou* or inch mouth in order to determine the death and life, good and evil auspices of the five viscera and six bowels. What does this mean?

Answer: The inch mouth is the great meeting of all the vessels located at the stirring vessel of the hand *tai yin*. When a person exhales once, [the contents of] the vessels move three inches. One inhalation, the vessels move [another] three inches. [One] exhalation and [one] inhalation establish [one] respiration [during which] the vessels move six inches. In humans, in one day and one night, there are 13,500 respirations, [during which the contents of] the vessels move 50 circuits around the body [in the time it takes for] water to drip downward 100 markings [on the water clock]. The constructive and defensive move [during] the yang 25 circuits, while they move also 25 circuits during the yin. This makes up one cycle. Therefore, [after] 50 circuits [the

---

[1] Stirring vessels refer to palpable arterial pulses.

contents of the vessels] return to meet at the hand *tai yin*. [Thus,] the inch mouth is the beginning and end of the five viscera and six bowels, and hence the method is to choose the inch mouth.

Two

Difficulty Two says: The pulse[2] has a cubit and an inch. What does this mean?

Answer: The cubit and inch are the great, important meetings of the vessels. From the bar to Cubit [Marsh, *i.e.*, *Chi Ze*, LI 11] is a cubit on the inner [side of the forearm]. It is the place where yin is treated [or dealt with]. From the bar to the Fish's [Belly, *i.e.*, the proximal margin of the thenar eminence] is the inch mouth. It is the place where yang is treated. Therefore, [the bar] separates the inch to make the cubit, [while it] separates the cubit to make the inch. Thus yin is obtained within the one inch of the cubit, [while] yang is obtained inside the nine *fen* of the inch. Cubit and inch [from] beginning to end is one inch, nine *fen*. Therefore, it is called the cubit and the inch.

---

[2] The word *mai* means both pulse and vessels. Unschuld solves this dilemma by translating this word as "[the movement within] the vessels."

Three

Difficulty Three says: The pulses can be greatly excessive or they may not reach. One may have yin and yang seizing each other, turnover, or spillage, bar or block. What does this mean?

Answer: In front of the bar is where yang stirs. The pulse seen in those nine *fen* is floating. [If extending] beyond [these nine *fen*], this is called greatly excessive. If vacuous, this is called not reaching. If it continues up the Fish's [Belly], this is spillage. This is made by external bar and internal block. This means yin is seizing the vessels. Behind the bar is where yin stirs. The pulse seen within this one inch is sunken. If [extending] beyond [this area], this is called greatly excessive. If vacuous, it is called not reaching. If it extends into the cubit, this is turnover. It is made by internal bar and external block. This means yang is seizing the vessels. Therefore, one speaks of turnover and spillage. These are the [so-called] true visceral pulses.

[Even] if the person is not diseased, this is [*i.e.*, means] death.[3]

---

[3] These pulses indicate death because they are signs that yin and yang have separated and are no longer inter-promoting and inter-restraining.

Four

Difficulty Four says: The pulses have the method of yin and yang. What does this mean?

Answer: Exhalation exits from the heart and lungs, while inhalation enters the kidneys and liver. Between inhalation and exhalation, the spleen receives grains and flavors. Its pulse is located in the center. Floating is yang and sunken is yin. This is what is called yin and yang.

The heart and lung [pulses] are both floating. How can one distinguish them?

Answer: Floating and greatly scattered [corresponds to] the heart. Floating, short, and astringent [corresponds to] the lungs.[4]

---

[4] Floating and scattered I take to mean so large or wide as to be without clearly defined edges. Floating, short, and astringent, I take to mean narrow with very well defined edges. In this case, I choose to translate *se* as astringent rather than as choppy.

If both the kidneys and liver are sunken, how can one distinguish them?

Answer: Confined and long [corresponds to] the liver. Press and soggy, lift the fingers and it comes replete [corresponds to] the kidneys. The spleen is the central islet. Therefore, its pulse is located in the middle. This is the method of yin and yang.

The pulse may have one yin and one yang, one yin and two yang, [or] one yin and three yang. [Or] it may have one yang and one yin, one yang and two yin, [or] one yang and three yin. Does this saying [mean] the inch mouth has six pulses all stirring [at the same time]?

Answer: This saying does not [mean] the six pulses are all stirring [at the same time]. This speaks of [or means] the floating and sunken, long, short, slippery, and choppy [pulses]. Floating is yang, slippery is yang, and long is yang. Sunken is yin, short is yin, and choppy is yin. Thus, when one speaks of one yin and one yang, it means the pulse comes sunken and slippery. One yin and two yang means the pulse comes sunken, slippery, and long. One yin and three yang, means the pulse comes floating, slippery, and long [but also] once in a while sunken. What is spoken of as one yang and one yin means the pulse comes floating and choppy. One yang and two yin, means the pulse comes long, sunken, and choppy. One yang and three yin means the pulse comes sunken, choppy, and short [but also] once in a while floating. In each [case], depending on which channel it is in, one knows [whether] the disease is [proceeding] counterflow or correctly.[5]

---

[5] *Ni* and *shun* literally mean counterflow and correct flow, but also mean ominous and auspicious in terms of prognosis.

Five

Difficulty Five says: The pulses have light and heavy. What does this mean?

Answer: First, hold the pulse. As heavy as three beans and obtained [at the level of] the skin and hair, this is the lung section.[6] As heavy as six beans and obtained [at the level of] the blood vessels, this is the heart section. As heavy as nine beans and obtained [at the level of] the muscles and flesh, this is the spleen section. As heavy as 12 beans and level with the sinews, this is the liver section. [If one] presses all the way to the bone, and lets up the fingers [until one feels] a fast [flowing again], this is the kidney section. Thus one speaks of light and heavy [in terms of the pulse].

---

[6] Skin and hair is a compound term which really only means skin.

Six

Difficulty Six says: The pulses have yin exuberance and yang vacuity and yang exuberance and yin vacuity. What does this mean?

Answer: If floating [*i.e.*, the superficial level of the pulse] is decreased and small, while sunken [or the deep level of the pulse] is replete and large, this is what is said to be yin exuberance, yang vacuity. If sunken is decreased and small, while floating is replete and large, this is what is said to be yang exuberance and yin vacuity. This is what is meant by yin and yang vacuity and repletion.

Seven

Difficulty Seven says: The [*Nei*] *Jing (Inner Classic)*[7] says the arrival of the *shao yang* may be large or small, short or long. The arrival of the *yang ming* is floating, large, and short. The arrival of the *tai yang* is surging, large, and long. The arrival of the *tai yin* is tight, large, and long. The arrival of the *shao yin* is tight, fine, and faint. And the arrival of the *jue yin* is sunken, short, and heavy. Are all six of these level [*i.e.*, normal] pulses or are they diseased pulses?

Answer: All these are king pulses.[8]

During which months and on what days is their qi king?

---

[7] From this point on, all references to *The Classic* mean the *Nei Jing*.

[8] This means that these pulses correspond to climatic divisions of time describing the waxing of qi in these various vessels. As such, they are normal, not diseased pulses.

Answer: After the winter solstice, [during the first subsequent] *jia zi* [term],[9] *shao yang* is king. From the next *jia zi*, *yang ming* is king. From the next *jia zi*, *tai yang* is king. From the next *jia zi*, *tai yin* is king. From the next *jia zi*, *shao yin* is king. From the next *jia zi*, *jue yin* is king. Each is king for 60 days. Six [times] six [makes] 360 days, thus producing one year. These are the great essentials of the three yin and three yang king times and days.

---

[9] One *jia zi* term means a 60 day cycle.

Eight

Difficulty Eight says: The inch mouth pulse [may be] level [*i.e.*, normal, and still there may be] death. What does this mean?

Answer: All 12 channel pulses are tied to the origin of living qi. What is spoken of as the origin of living qi is the root of the 12 channels. It is the moving qi between the kidneys. This is the root of the five viscera and six bowels, the root of the 12 channels and their pulses, the gate of inhalation and exhalation, and the origin of the three burners. Another name is the spirit guarding against evils. Therefore, qi is a person's root. If the root is cut, the stalks and leaves must wither. If the inch mouth pulse is level and there is death, this can only be that the living qi is severed [or cut off] internally.

Nine

Difficulty Nine says: How can one distinguish diseases in the viscera and the bowels?

Answer: Rapid [and the disease] is in the bowels. Slow [and the disease] is in the viscera. Rapidity is due to heat. Slowness is due to cold. All yang [conditions] are made by heat. All yin [conditions] are made by cold. Thereby can one distinguish diseases of the viscera and the bowels.

Ten

Difficulty Ten says: Each pulse has 10 changes. What does this mean?

Answer: This has to do with the concepts of the five evils, hardness and softness, and mutual interference. For example, if the heart pulse is very tense, liver evils have entered the heart. If the heart pulse is slightly tense, gallbladder evils have entered the small intestine. If the heart pulse is very large, heart evils have entered the heart itself. If the heart pulse is slightly large, small intestine evils have entered the small intestine itself. If the heart pulse is very moderate [meaning slightly slow, so, in this case, very slow], spleen evils have entered the heart. If the heart pulse is slightly moderate [i.e., slightly slow], stomach evils have entered the small intestine. If the heart pulse is very choppy, lung evils have entered the heart. If the heart pulse is slightly choppy, large intestine evils have entered the small intestine. If the heart pulse is very sunken, kidney evils have entered the heart. If the heart pulse is slightly sunken, bladder evils have entered the small intestine. [Thus,] the five viscera each have their hard and

soft evils, and hence each pulse [position] may
undergo 10 changes.

Eleven

Difficulty Eleven says: *The Classic* says if the pulse does not fill 50 stirrings [*i.e.*, beats] but stops once, one viscus is without qi. What does this mean?

Answer: A person's inhalation follows yin and enters, while exhalation is due to yang and exits. If inhalation is not able to reach the kidneys but reaches the liver and then returns, we know that one viscus is without qi and that it is the kidney qi which is first exhausted.

Twelve

Difficulty Twelve says: *The Classic* says that, if the five visceral pulses are already severed internally, it is contrary [*i.e.*, wrong] to use needles to make replete the external. If the five visceral pulses are already severed externally, it is contrary to use needles to make replete the interior. How can one distinguish between internal and external severance?

Answer: If the five visceral pulses are already severed internally, [this means that] the kidney and liver vessels are severed internally. [In that case,] the doctor [acts] contrarily if he supplements the heart and lungs. If the five visceral pulses are already severed externally, [this means that] the heart and lung vessels are severed externally. [In that case,] the doctor [acts] contrarily if he supplements the kidneys and liver. If yang is severed and one supplements yin or if yin is severed and one supplements yang, this is what is called repleting repletion and [making] vacuous vacuity. [This causes] detriment to what is insufficient and boosts what is already surplus. If, like this, one dies, it is the doctor who killed him.

Thirteen

Difficulty Thirteen says: *The Classic* says, if one sees [a person's] color [*i.e.*, facial complexion] and cannot obtain the [corresponding] pulse but contrarily obtains a pulse [indicating] mutual vanquishment, [the person will] die. If one obtains a pulse of mutual engenderment, the disease will end on its own. [Therefore, a person's] color and pulse should be compared for mutual correspondence, but how is this done?

Answer: The five viscera have five colors, each of which can be seen on the face. These should also correspond to the [pulse at] the inch mouth and [the condition of the skin on] the inside [*i.e.*, ventral surface of] the cubit.

For example, if the color [of the facial complexion] is green, the pulse should be bowstring[10] and tense. If the color is red, the

___

[10] Wiseman recommends stringlike for *xian*. However, stringlike does not necessarily imply the quality of tautness this pulse image describes. Therefore, I prefer the term bowstring, which is what the Chinese character originally described.

pulse should be floating, large, and scattered.[11]
If the color is yellow, the pulse should be
medium, moderate [*i.e.*, slightly slow], and
large. If the color is white, the pulse should be
floating, choppy[12], and short. If the color is
black, the pulse should be sunken, soggy[13], and
slippery. This is what is meant by the saying
that the color and pulse should mutually
correspond.

---

[11] I believe that the word scattered when applied to the
pulse means a pulse without discernible edges.

[12] Wiseman recommends rough pulse for *se mai*. In a
previous glossary, *A Glossary of Chinese Medical Terms and
Acupuncture Points*, Paradigm Press, Brookline, MA, 1995,
he recommended choppy. We have decided to retain
choppy since this is what most Western practitioners use
and what we use in the majority of our books.

[13] For me, the soggy pulse means a pulse which is
floating, fine, and forceless. Since the author of the *Nan
Jing* says the pulse is both sunken and soggy, he may
mean that it is fine and forceless, although this is not
absolutely clear.

If the pulse is rapid, the skin on the inside of the cubit should also be rapid.[14] If the pulse is tense, the cubit skin should also be tense. If the pulse is moderate, the cubit skin should also be moderate.[15] If the pulse is choppy, the cubit skin should also be choppy [i.e., rough]. If the pulse is slippery, the cubit skin should also be slippery.

[Likewise,] the five viscera each have a sound, color, smell, flavor and the inch mouth and inside cubit should mutually correspond [with these respectively]. If there is no correspondence, there is disease. For example, if the color is green and the pulse is floating, choppy, and short or it is large and moderate, this is mutual

---

[14] It is hard to understand how skin can feel "rapid." Various commentators have tried to reconcile what may simply be a typographical error. Ding De-yong says the skin is hot, while Xu Da-chun suspects there is a typo.

[15] Wiseman translates the word *huan* as moderate when describing the pulse, in which case, it implies that the pulse is slightly slow. However, the word might also be translated as relaxed. Therefore, when the pulse is slightly slow, the cubit skin should feel relaxed.

vanquishment. If it is floating, large, and scattered or it is small [meaning fine] and slippery, this is mutual engenderment.

The Classic says the inferior worker knows one [sign], the medium worker knows two [signs], [while] the superior worker knows three [signs]. The superior worker makes whole nine [out of] ten [patients]. The medium worker makes whole eight out of ten. The inferior worker makes whole six out of ten. Thus it is said.

Fourteen

Difficulty Fourteen says: The pulse may have detriment and arrival. What does this mean?

Answer: Arrival of the pulse [means that for] one exhalation, two [beats] arrive. This is called level [or normal]. If three [beats] arrive, this is called departure from regular.[16] If four arrive, this is called loss of essence. If five arrive, this is called death. If six arrive, this is called severing of one's destiny.[17] These are the arrivals of the pulse.[18]

How is detriment called?

One exhalation, one arrival is called departure from regular. Two exhalations, one arrival is called loss of essence. Three exhalations, one

---

[16] It is interesting to note that the word for regular used here is *jing*, also the word for channel.

[17] The word *ming* means life's destiny, not simply life itself.

[18] Based on the foregoing description, it appears that arrival of the pulse describes rapid pulses.

arrival is called death. And four exhalations and one arrival is called severed destiny. These are the detriments of the pulse.[19]

Arrival of the pulse goes from lower [to upper]. Detriment of the pulse goes from upper [to] lower.[20]

What disease is signaled by detriment of the pulse?

Answer: One detriment [*i.e.*, the first stage of detriment], is detriment of the skin and hair. The skin is gathered [*i.e.*, wrinkled] and the hair is missing [*i.e.*, falling]. The second detriment is detriment of the blood vessels. The blood vessels are vacuous and scanty and are not able to construct the five viscera and six bowels. The third detriment is detriment of the muscles and flesh. The muscles and flesh are dispersed and emaciated. Food and drink are not able to make

---

[19] Based on the foregoing description, it appears that detriment of the pulse describes slow pulses.

[20] Lower and upper means lower and upper viscera.

the muscles and skin. The fourth detriment is detriment of the sinews. The sinews are relaxed [*i.e.*, slack] and not able to contract and take hold. The fifth detriment is detriment of the bones. The bones are wilted and one is not able to rise from bed. Contrary [or opposite to this] is arrival resulting in disease. [Therefore, if the disease] proceeds from above to below, there is death when bone wilting [causes] inability to arise from bed. [If the disease] proceeds from below to above, there is death when the skin becomes gathered and the hair is missing.

What are the methods for treating detriment?

Answer: For detriment of the lungs, boost its qi. For detriment of the heart, regulate the constructive and defensive. For detriment of the spleen, regulate its food and drink, [insuring] suitable cold and warmth. For detriment of the liver, moderate [*i.e.*, relax] the center. For detriment of the kidneys, boost their essence. These are the methods of treating detriment.

The pulse may have two arrivals in one exhalation and two arrivals in one inhalation. It may have three arrivals in one exhalation and three arrivals in one inhalation. It may have four arrivals in one exhalation and four arrivals in one inhalation. It may have five arrivals in one exhalation and five arrivals in one inhalation. It may have six arrivals in one exhalation and six arrivals in one inhalation. It may have one arrival in one exhalation and one arrival in one inhalation. It may have one arrival in two exhalations and one arrival in two inhalations. Or it may have two arrivals in an exhalation and inhalation. When the pulse comes like this, how can one distinguish their diseases?

Answer: If the pulse comes with two arrivals in one exhalation and two arrivals in one inhalation, not larger [*i.e.*, more], not smaller [*i.e.*, less, this is] called level [or normal]. If there are three arrivals in one exhalation and three arrivals in one inhalation, this is just [the beginning of] obtaining a disease. If in front, the pulse is large, while behind, it is small, there is headache and dizziness.[21] If in front, [the pulse

---

[21] In front means in front of the bar or the inch position. Behind means behind the bar or the cubit position.

is] small and behind, it is large, there is chest fullness and shortness of qi [*i.e.*, shortness of breath]. If there is four arrivals in one exhalation and four arrivals in one inhalation, the disease is tending towards [or becoming] severe. If the pulse is surging and large, there is bitterness, vexation, and fullness. If sunken and fine, there is abdominal and middle pain. If slippery, there is damage [due to] heat. If choppy, there is mist and dew in the center. If there are five arrivals in one exhalation and five arrivals in one inhalation, the person must be encumbered [*i.e.*, critical]. If sunken and fine, [the disease will] increase at night. If floating and large, it will increase during the day. If neither large nor small, even though encumbered, [the patient] can be treated. If either large or small, this makes treatment difficult. If there are six arrivals in one exhalation and six arrivals in one inhalation, this makes for a death pulse. If sunken and fine, [the patient will] die at night. If floating and large, they will die during the day.

One exhalation, one arrival, one inhalation, one arrival, this is called detriment. The person may still be able to move [*i.e.*, walk] but should remain in bed. The reason for this is because both the qi and blood are insufficient. Two exhalations, one arrival, two inhalations, one arrival, this is called no *hun* [*i.e.*, the ethereal soul]. If there is no *hun*, there must be death. If the person is still able to move, this is called moving [*i.e.*, walking] corpse. If the upper position [*i.e.*, the inch] has a pulse but there is no pulse in the lower position [*i.e.*, the cubit], the person must vomit. If there is no vomiting, there is death. If there is no pulse in the upper position but the lower position has a pulse, even though [the condition is] critical, [the patient] is not able to be harmed. The reason for this is because a person's having a cubit [pulse] is like a tree having a root. Although the branches and leaves are withered, the root can live by itself. [Likewise,] the pulse has its root. In people, it is the source qi. Therefore, one knows [there is] no death.

Fifteen

Difficulty Fifteen says: *The Classic* says that in the spring, the pulse is bowstring. In summer, the pulse is hook[-like]. In autumn, the pulse is hair[-like]. While in winter, it is stone[-like]. Are these king pulses or are they disease pulses?

Answer: Bowstring, hook[-like], hair[-like], and stone[-like] are the pulses of the four times [or seasons]. In spring, the pulse is bowstring because [this season corresponds to] the liver, the east, and wood. [During this time,] the tens of thousands of things are born. [Trees] do not [yet] have branches and leaves. Therefore, when the pulse comes, it is soggy,[22] weak, and long.[23] Thus it is called bowstring.

---

[22] *Ru*, soggy, is the proper name of an individual pulse image, in which case it means floating, fine, and forceless. Here I believe the author only means to imply the pulse is forceless.

[23] The word long here does not imply the long pulse but only that one can feel the longitudinality of the pulse under their fingers.

In summer, the pulse is hook[-like] because [this season corresponds to] the heart, the south, and fire. [During this season,] the tens of thousands of things are fully grown. The branches hang down and the leaves spread, curving downward like hooks. Thus the pulse comes racing and departs slowly. Therefore, it is called hook [-like].

In autumn, the pulse is hair[-like] because [this season corresponds to] the lungs, the west, and metal. [During this season,] the tens of thousands of things are finished. Grass, trees, flowers, and leaves fall and are missing. Only the branches remain resembling fine hairs. Thus, when the pulse comes, it is soft, vacuous, and floating. Therefore, it is called hair[-like].

In winter, the pulse is stone[-like] because [this season corresponds to] the kidneys, north, and water. [During this season,] the tens of thousands of things are stored. When winter is exuberant [*i.e.*, at its peak], water congeals like stone. Thus, when the pulse comes, it is sunken, soggy, and slippery. Therefore, it is called stone [-like]. These are the pulses of the four seasons.

What if they are different [than this]?

Answer: In spring, the pulse should be
bowstring. Contrary [to this] makes for disease.

What does contrary mean?

Answer: If the qi comes replete and strong, this
is called greatly excessive and the disease is in
the external. If the qi comes vacuous and faint,
this is called not reaching. The disease is in the
internal. If the qi comes serene and whispering,
like elm leaves [in a light breeze], this is called
level [or normal]. [If the pulse comes]
increasingly replete and slippery, like long
canes, this is called diseased. [If it comes] tense,
sturdy, and increasingly strong, like a new
bowstring, this is called death. In spring, a pulse
which is slightly bowstring is called level. If it is
mostly bowstring and the stomach qi is scanty,
this is called diseased. However, bowstring with
no stomach qi is called death. In spring, the
stomach qi is the root.

In summer, the pulse is hook[-like]. Contrary to this makes for disease. What does contrary mean [here]?

Answer: If the qi comes replete and strong, this is called greatly excessive and disease is in the external. If the qi comes vacuous and faint, this is called not reaching. [In that case,] disease is in the internal. If the pulse comes continuously without break like links of *lang gan* [a type of jade], this is called level. If it comes increasingly rapidly, like chickens lifting their feet, this is called diseased. If in front [of the bar], it is curved but behind, it is abiding [straightly as it should and, thus, is] like a hook holding a belt, this is called death. In summer, if the pulse is slightly hooked, this is called level. If mostly hooked with scanty stomach qi, this is called diseased. However, if it is hooked with no stomach qi, this is called death. In summer, the stomach qi is the root.

The autumn pulse is hair[-like]. Contrary [to this] makes for disease. What does this contrary mean?

Answer: If the qi comes replete and strong, this is called greatly excessive and the disease is in the external. If the qi comes vacuous and faint, this is called not reaching and the disease is in the internal. If the pulse comes luxuriantly like the canopy of a carriage and, if pressing it becomes increasingly large, this is called level. [If the pulse remains] neither above nor below [the bar but flaps] like a chicken's wing, this is called diseased. If, when pressed, it is like a loose rope or like hair blown by the wind, this is called death. If the autumn pulse is slightly hair [-like], this is called level. If it is mostly hair [-like] with scanty stomach qi, this is called diseased. However, if it is hair[-like] with no stomach qi, this is called death. In autumn, the stomach qi is the root.

Winter's pulse is stone[-like]. Contrary [to this] makes for disease. What does this contrary mean?

Answer: If the qi comes replete and strong, this is called greatly excessive and the disease is in the external. If the qi comes vacuous and faint, this is called not reaching and the disease is in the internal. If the pulse comes above large and below sharply, yet soggy and slippery like a sparrow's beak, this is called level. If continuously pecking and slightly curved in the center, this is called diseased. If it comes like an unknotted rope and departs like a stone pellet, this is called death. If the winter pulse is slightly stone[-like], this is called level. If it is mostly stone[-like] with scanty stomach qi, this is called diseased. However, if it is stone[-like] with no stomach qi, this is called death. In winter, the stomach qi is the root. The stomach is the sea of water and grains. It governs the endowment of the four times [or seasons. Hence] the stomach qi is root of all these. These are what are called changes [in the pulses and their corresponding] diseases of the four times. They are the essence for understanding life and death.

The spleen is the central islet. Its levelness and harmony [*i.e.*, its harmonious normality] cannot be seen [in the pulse. Only] its decline manifests [in the pulse]. If it comes like a sparrow pecking or like water dripping downward, this is how spleen decline manifests [in the pulse].

Sixteen

Difficulty Sixteen says: The pulse has three positions and nine indicators, it has yin and yang, it has light and heavy [pressure], and it has 60 chief [images]. A single pulse may change due to the four times [or seasons]. The distance from the sages is long and far, and [today] everyone has their own method. How can one distinguish [among these]?

Answer: Each disease has internal and external symptoms.

What evidence do diseases create?

Answer: For example, if one obtains the liver pulse, externally, [there should be] these symptoms: a predilection for cleanliness, a greenish color [to the facial complexion], and a predilection to anger. Internally, [there should be] these symptoms: stirring qi to the left of the navel which [feels] hard and painful to pressure. Its diseases: fullness of the four limbs, [urinary] block and strangury, and difficult urination and defecation. If one has these, there is liver [disease]. If one does not have these, then there is no [liver disease].

As [another] example, if one obtains the heart pulse, the external symptoms [of heart viscus disease] are a red color [to the facial complexion], dry mouth, a liking for laughter. Its internal symptoms are stirring qi above the navel which is hard and painful when pressed. Its diseases: heart vexation, heart pain, heat in the center of the palms, and nausea. If one has these, there is heart [disease]. If one does not have these, there is no [heart disease].

Yet [another] example, if one obtains the spleen pulse, the external symptoms [of spleen disease] are a yellow color [to the facial complexion] and a predilection for thinking. Internal symptoms include a stirring qi at the navel which is hard and painful when pressed. Its diseases: abdominal distention and fullness, non-dispersion of food, bodily heaviness, joint pain, fatigue, a desire to lie down, and lack of control over the four limbs. If one has these, there is spleen [disease]. If one does not have these, there is no [spleen disease].

Again, if one obtains the lung pulse, the external symptoms [of lung disease] are a white color [to the facial complexion], a tendency to sneeze, grief, sorrow, no happiness, and desire to cry. The internal symptom [of lung disease] is a stirring qi to the right of the navel which is hard and painful with pressure. Its diseases include cough and shivering with cold and heat. If one has these, there is lung [disease]. If one does not have these, there is no [lung disease].

And [finally], if one obtains the kidney pulse, the external symptoms [of kidney disease] are a black color [to the facial complexion], a tendency to fear, and blowing [*i.e.*, flatulence]. Internal symptoms include a stirring qi below the navel which is hard and painful with pressure. Its diseases include counterflow qi, lower abdominal cramping and pain, diarrhea with tenesmus, and foot and shin coldness and counterflow. If one has these, there is kidney [disease]. If one does not have these, there is no [kidney disease].

Seventeen

Difficulty Seventeen says: *The Classic* says diseased [persons] may die or they may automatically heal without treatment. Or they may continue [to be ill for] years and months without cease. By feeling the pulse, can one know who will live and who will die, who will exist and who will perish?

Answer: One can know this completely. If one examines a diseased [person] who shuts his eyes and has no desire to see people, the pulse one should obtain is the liver pulse, strong, tense, and long. If, contrarily, one obtains the lung pulse, floating, short, and choppy, this is death. If the diseased [person] open their eyes, is thirsty, and below their heart is hard, the pulse obtained should be tight, replete, and rapid. If, contrarily, [the pulse] obtained is sunken, choppy, and faint, this is death. If the diseased [person] spits blood and there is nasal congestion and spontaneous ejection of blood [*i.e.*, epistaxis], the pulse should be sunken and fine. If, contrarily, it is floating, large, and hard, this is death. If the diseased [person] speaks incoherently and utters nonsense, their body should have heat and their pulse should be surging and large. If, contrarily, there is inversion chilling of the hands and feet and the pulse is sunken, fine, and faint, this is death. If the diseased [person's] abdomen is enlarged and they have diarrhea, their pulse should be faint, fine, and choppy. If, contrarily, it is tight, large, and slippery, this is death.

Eighteen

Difficulty Eighteen says: The pulse has three positions, and [each] position has four channels. The hand has *tai yin* and *yang ming* and the foot has *tai yang* and *shao yin*. These make up the upper and lower positions. What does this mean?

Answer: The hand *tai yin* and *yang ming* are metal. The foot *shao yin* and *tai yang* are water. Metal engenders water. Water flows and moves downward and is unable to ascend. Therefore, [these two] are located in the lower position. The foot *jue yin* and *shao yang* are wood. They engender hand *tai yang* and *shao yin* fire. Fire flames and moves upward and is not able to descend. Therefore, these make up the upper position. The hand heart ruler is *shao yang* fire. It engenders foot *tai yin* and *yang ming* earth. Earth governs the central palace. Therefore, they are located in the middle position. All of this is five phase child-mother mutual engenderment and nourishment.

The pulse has three positions and nine indicators. What [diseases] rule each of these?

Answer: The three positions are the inch, bar, and cubit. The nine indicators are floating, medium, and sunken.[24] The upper position is modeled on heaven. It is governed by diseases of the chest up to the head. The middle position is modeled on humanity. It is governed by diseases from the diaphragm down to the navel. The lower position is modeled on earth. It is governed by diseases from the navel down to the feet.

If a diseased person has deep, stagnant, enduring accumulations and gatherings, can one feel the pulse and know this?

Answer: You examine a diseased [person and find] right rib-side accumulated qi and you obtain a bound lung pulse. A severely bound pulse and there are severe accumulations. If [only] slightly, the accumulations are slight.

---

[24] Because each of these three is likewise divided into three, there are nine indicators altogether, even though the text only names three.

If, on examination, you do not obtain a lung pulse but the right rib-side has accumulated qi, what then?

Answer: Although no lung pulse is seen, the right hand [pulse] should be sunken and deep-lying.

Is the method the same for external chronic diseases?

Answer: Bound [means that] the pulse stops once in a while when departing. [This stop] is without constant number [*i.e.*, the intervals between such pauses are irregularly intermittent]. This is what is called the bound [pulse]. Deep-lying [means that] the pulse moves under the sinews. Floating [means that] the pulse moves above where the flesh is located. [No matter whether the disease is located] on the left or on the right, in the exterior or in the interior, the method is like this.

For example, the pulse may be bound and deeply lying, yet internally there are no accumulations and gatherings; or the pulse may be floating and bound yet externally there are no chronic diseases. [It is also possible that] one may have accumulations and gatherings and the pulse is not bound or deep-lying; or one may have chronic [external] disease and the pulse is not floating. [In those cases,] the pulse does not correspond to the disease and the disease does not correspond to the pulse. This is a deadly [i.e., fatal] disease.

Nineteen

Difficulty Nineteen says: *The Classic* says the pulse may be counterflowing [*i.e.*, inauspicious] or correctly flowing [*i.e.*, auspicious. Likewise,] men and women have what is usual [or normal] and what is contrary. What does this mean?

Answer: Males are born in the *yin* [month].[25] *Yin* is wood and yang. Females are born in the *shen* [month]. *Shen* is metal and yin.[26] Therefore, a male's pulse is located above the bar [*i.e.*, is largest and strongest above the bar]. A female's pulse is located below the bar. [Therefore,] a male's cubit pulse should regularly be weak, while a female's cubit pulse should regularly be exuberant. This is what is normal. Contrarily, a man may have a woman's pulse, and a woman may have a man's pulse.

What disease is known by this?

---

[25] *Yin* here refers to one of the 12 terrestrial branches.

[26] This passage has nothing to do with what actual month a person is born in. It is based on abstruse numerological ideas about differences in internal development between men and women.

Answer: A man's obtaining a woman's pulse is due to insufficiency, and the disease is internal. If obtained on the left, the disease is on the left. If obtained on the right, the disease is on the right. Following the [specific] pulse [images], one can determine [the specific disease]. A female's obtaining a male's pulse is due to great excess and disease is located in the four extremities. If obtained on the left, the disease is on the left. If obtained on the right, the disease is on the right. Following the [specific] pulse [images], one can determine [the specific disease]. This is what is meant [by these terms].

Twenty

Difficulty Twenty says: *The Classic* says the pulses may be deep-lying and concealed. Deep-lying and concealed pertain to which viscera when it speaks of deep-lying and concealed?

Answer: [This saying] implies that yin and yang may mutually seize [each other's position] and mutually hide [in one another. A yin] pulse should abide in a yin position. If, contrarily, a yang pulse is seen, this is due to yang seizing yin. If that pulse is sometimes sunken, choppy, and short, it is said that yin is deeply lying within yang. [A yang] pulse should abide in a yang position. If, contrarily, a yin pulse is seen, this is due to yin seizing yang. If that pulse is sometimes floating, slippery, and long, this is called yang deeply lying within yin. Double yang [results in] mania, while double yin [results in] epilepsy. If yang deserts, one sees ghosts. If yin deserts, ones eyes go blind.

Twenty-one

Difficulty Twenty-one says: *The Classic* says if a person's body is diseased but their pulse is not diseased, this is called life. If the pulse is diseased but their body is not diseased, this is called death. What does this mean?

Answer: If a person's body is diseased but their pulse is not diseased, that does not [mean] there is no disease. It means that the number of respirations does not correspond to the number of pulses [*i.e.*, the speed of the pulse]. This is a great [or important] law.[27]

---

[27] This difficulty is pretty opaque, and many Chinese scholars have advanced radically different explanations of it. According to Ding De-yong, this lack of correspondence between the physical symptoms and the pulse has to do with the two viscera which control the movement of the qi and blood, the heart and lungs. If the pulse is diseased but the body is not diseased, this suggests a heart-lung disease, an ominous condition. If the body is diseased but the pulse is not, this suggests a spleen, liver, and/or kidney disease. However, since the heart and lungs are not yet affected, recovery is possible.

Twenty-two

Difficulty Twenty-two says: *The Classic* says the vessels may be stirred or there may be the engenderment of disease. One vessel may thus become altered by two [kinds of] disease. How is this?

Answer: [When] *The Classic* says there may be stirring, this [refers to stirring of] the qi. [When it says] there may be the engenderment of disease, this [refers to disease within the] blood. If evils exist in the qi [division], the qi is stirred. If these evils exist [or enter] into the blood [division], the blood is where disease will be engendered. It is the qi which governs shining [*i.e.*, fuming and steaming], while the blood governs moistening. If the qi lingers and does not move, the qi first becomes diseased. If the blood [subsequently] becomes obstructed and does not moisten, then the blood becomes diseased after. Therefore, first there is stirring and later there is engenderment [of disease].[28]

---

[28] This difficulty is not very clear and has produced numerous differing interpretations amongst commentators. It seems to me to be talking about the

Twenty-three

Difficulty Twenty-three says: Do you know anything about the measurements of the hand and foot three yin and three yang [channels]?

Answer: The hand three yang vessels go from the hand and arrive at the head. They are five cubits long. Five [cubits times] six adds up to three *chang*. The hand three yin vessels go from the hand and arrive at the center of the chest. They are three cubits and five inches long. Three [cubits times] six[29] adds up to one *chang* and eight cubits. Five [cubits times] six [equals] three cubits. Added together, [this gives] two *chang* and one cubit. The foot three yang vessels go from the feet and arrive at the head. They are eight cubits long. Six [times] eight [cubits equal] four *chang* and eight cubits. The foot three yin vessels go from the feet and arrive at the chest.

---

progression from functional to organic diseases, suggesting that symptoms of functional disease manifest before organic disease.

[29] There are three hand yang vessels which are found on each of two sides. Therefore, in terms of total length, there are six hand yang channels.

They are six cubits and five inches long. Six
[cubits times] six [equals] three *chang* and six
cubits. Five [inches times] six [equals] three
cubits. [So] altogether they are three *chang* and
nine cubits. A person [also] has two foot *qiao*
vessels. These go from the feet and arrive at the
eyes. They are seven cubits and five inches long.
Two [times] seven [equals] one *chang* and four
cubits. Two [times] five [inches equals] one
cubit. [So] altogether they are one *chang* and five
cubits. [As for] the governing vessel and the
conception vessel, each is four cubits and five
inches long. Two [times] four [cubits equals]
eight cubits. Two [times] five [inches equals]
one cubit. [So] altogether they are nine cubits.
All the vessels together are 16 *chang* and two
cubits long. These are the numbers of the long
and short [*i.e.*, these are the lengths] of the 12
channel vessels.

There are 12 channel vessels and 15 network
vessels. Where do these start and where do they
end?

Answer: The channel vessels move the qi and
blood and connect yin and yang in order to

[provide] construction [*i.e.*, nourishment] to the body. The [qi and blood] begin in the middle burner and pour into the hand *tai yin* and *yang ming*. The [hand] *yang ming* pours into the foot *yang ming* and *tai yin*. The [foot] *tai yin* pours into the hand *shao yin* and *tai yang*. The [hand] *tai yang* pours into the foot *tai yang* and *shao yin*. The [foot] *shao yin* pours into the heart governor and [hand] *shao yang*. The [hand] *shao yang* pours into the foot *shao yang* and *jue yin*. The [foot] *jue yin* returns in a circle to pour into the hand *tai yin*.

There are 15 divergent network vessels which all carry on [back over and over again] to their origin, like a ring without an end, transmitting mutually [one to the next] and irrigating, daily presenting at the inch mouth and human prognosis. Therefore, [all] the hundreds of diseases and life and death can be determined [at the inch mouth and human prognosis].

The Classic states that a clear understanding of end and beginning can be established. What does this mean?

Answer: End and beginning can be recorded [*i.e.*, inferred] from the pulses. Yin and yang qi connect with the inch mouth and human prognosis [each] morning.[30] This is like a ring without end. This is what is called the beginning. [In terms of] the end, if the three yin and three yang vessels are severed, severance leads to death. Each death [*i.e.*, each critical situation due to the severance of a particular vessel] has its form [or bodily symptoms]. This is what is called the end.

---

[30] In this case, the inch mouth is yin and the human prognosis is yang.

Twenty-four

Difficulty Twenty-four says: What are the indicators if the hand and foot three yin and three yang has already been severed? Can one know favorable and unfavorable or not?

Answer: If the foot *shao yin* is severed, this leads to bone withering. The *shao yin* is the pulse of winter. It moves deep-lying and warms the bones and marrow. Therefore, if the bones and marrow are not warmed, the flesh will not adhere to the bones. If the bones and the flesh do not mutually marry, the flesh will become soggy and shrink. If the flesh becomes soggy and shrinks, then the teeth will be long and withered. The hair will lose its moisture and shine. [If the hair has] no moisture and shine, first the bones [must have already] died. [In that case, the disease will become] severe on a *wu* day and death will come on a *ji* day.

If the foot *tai yin* is severed, this leads to its vessels not constructing the mouth and lips. The mouth and lips are the root of the muscles and flesh. If the vessels do not construct, the muscles and flesh are not glossy [i.e., smooth] and shiny.

If the muscles and flesh are not glossy and shiny, the flesh is full. If the flesh is full, the lips [curl] backwards.[31] If the lips [curl] backward, the flesh [must have] first died. [In that case, the disease will become] severe on *jia* days, and death will come on a *yi* day.

If the foot *jue yin* qi is severed, the sinews will contract, the testicles will be [with]drawn, and the tongue will curl [back]. The *jue yin* is the liver pulse, and the liver is the meeting of the sinews. The sinews gather in the yin organs and a network vessel [of the *jue yin* goes] to the root of the tongue. Therefore, if this vessel [gets] no construction, the sinews become contracted and tense. If the sinews become contracted and tense, the testicles and tongue are drawn. Hence, if the tongue curls [back] and the testicles contract, the sinews [must have] died first. [In that case, the disease will become] severe on *geng* days, and death will come on a *xin* day.

---

[31] Fullness of the flesh implies edematous swelling. Since the lips are also edematous, they extend outward and back.

If the hand *tai yin* qi is severed, the skin and hair will be scorched. The *tai yin* is the lungs. [The lungs] move the qi [which] warms the skin and hair. If the qi does not construct, the skin and hair are scorched. If skin and hair are scorched, fluids and humors depart. If fluids and humors depart, the skin joints are damaged. If the skin joints are damaged, the skin is withered and the hair is broken. [Therefore, when] the hair breaks, the hair [must] first have died. [In that case, the disease will become] severe on *bing* days, and death will come on a *ding* day.

If the hand *shao yin* qi is severed, the vessels will not flow freely. If the vessels do not flow freely, the blood will not flow. If the blood does not flow, the color and shininess [of the facial complexion] will depart. Therefore, the facial color is black like a pear [*i.e.*, a blackish yellow color]. [In that case,] the blood [must have] died first. [The disease will become] severe on *ren* days, and death will come on a *gui* day.

If the qi of all three yin [vessels] is severed, one's vision will become dizzy and turn and one's eyes will close. When one's eyes close, one loses one's mind [*i.e.*, becomes unconscious]. If one loses one's mind, the mind [must have] died first. When one has died, the eyes are closed.

If the qi of all six yang is severed, yin and yang mutually separate. When yin and yang mutually separate, the interstices [or pores] discharge. Then sweat is discharged, intermittently [the drops] large as pearl beads. These roll out but do not flow. [In that case,] the qi [must] first have died. [If this occurs at] dawn, death will come at sunset. [If this occurs at] sunset, death will come at dawn.

Twenty-five

Difficulty Twenty-five says: There are 12 channels and there are five viscera and six bowels making 11. What is this extra channel?

Answer: [In terms of this] one channel, the hand *shao yin* and heart governor are differentiated [into two separate] vessels. The heart governor and triple burner make an exterior and interior [pair]. Both have a name but no form. Therefore, one speaks of 12 channels.

Twenty-six

Difficulty Twenty-six says: There are 12 channels and 15 network vessels. This leaves three network vessels. What are these extra network vessels?

Answer: There is a yang network vessel, a yin network vessel, and a great network vessel of the spleen. The yang network vessel is the network vessel of the *yang qiao* [vessel], while the yin network vessel is the network vessel of the *yin qiao* [vessel]. Therefore, there are 15 network vessels.

Twenty-seven

Difficulty Twenty-seven says: The vessels
[also] have the extraordinary[32] channel eight
vessels that are not delimited by [*i.e.*, included
in] the 12 channels. What does this mean?

Answer: There is the *yang wei,* the *yin wei,* the
yang qiao, the *yin qiao,* the *chong,* the governing,
the conception, and the belt vessels. All these
eight vessels are not delimited by the channels.
Therefore, they are called the extraordinary
channel eight vessels.

The channels have 12 and the network vessels
have 15. Altogether, [this makes] 27 qi which
follow each other up and down. What [does it
mean that these eight] are alone and not
delimited by the channels?

Answer: The sages mapped out and con-
structed ditches and reservoirs, freeing the flow
and disinhibiting the water passageways in
order to be prepared for unusual [situations.

---

[32] Extraordinary means both single, *i.e.*, not paired, and
unusual.

However,] when heaven's rains descended, these ditches and reservoirs spilled over and were filled. In times like those, rain-floods rushed wildly, and even the ages were not able to restore their scheme. [Likewise,] when the network vessels are full and spill over, the channels are not able to detain [or contain this overflow].[33]

---

[33] The word *ju*, detain or restrain, used here is the same as the word translated as delimited in the original question. Thus there seems to be a play on words here. The eight extraordinary vessels are not contained or delimited by the 12 regular channels but fill with the overflow these 12 channels cannot detain or contain.

Twenty-eight

Difficulty Twenty-eight says: If the extra-ordinary channel eight vessels are not delimited by the 12 channels, from where do they arise and to where do they continue?

Answer: The governing vessel arises from the lower end [of the body's] transport [point, *i.e., Hui Yin*, CV 1]. It joins the interior of the spine and ascends to arrive at Wind Mansion (*Feng Fu*, GV 16), where it enters and homes to the brain. The conception vessel arises from below Central Pole (*Zhong Ji*, CV 3) from where it ascends to arrive at the edge of the [pubic] hair. It courses into the interior of the abdomen and ascends to Pass Head (*Guan Yuan*, CV 4) [eventually to] arrive at the throat. The *chong mai* arises at Qi Thoroughfare (*Qi Chong*, St 30). It joins the foot *yang ming* channel, moves above the navel, arrives in the center of the chest, and scatters. The *dai mai* arises from the last rib and then encircles the entire circumference of the body. The *yang qiao mai* arises within the heel, courses over the outside of the heel and moves upward to enter Wind Pool (*Feng Chi*, GB 20). The *yin qiao mai* also arises within the heel but courses over the inside of the heel, moves upward, and arrives at the throat, joining and linking with the *chong mai*. The *yang wei* and *yin wei* [vessels] are tied [like] a network with the body. When they spill over, [their contents mill about like] a herd and are not able to circulate and irrigate the other channels. Hence the *yang wei* arises where all the yang [channels] meet, while the *yin wei* arises where all the yin [channels] intersect.

This is like the sages' planning and creating ditches and reservoirs. When the ditches and reservoirs are full and spilling over, [this surplus] flows into deep lakes since [even] the sages were not able to detain this [and insure its continuous] free flow. Similarly, when a person's vessels are swollen and exuberant, [the surplus qi and blood] enters these eight vessels where they no [longer] circulate around because the 12 channels are not able to detain [or contain them]. If they receive evil qi [which mills about like] a herd, this may lead to swelling and heat. [In that case, use] a stone needle to spurt this out [by bleeding the affected vessel].

Twenty-nine

Difficulty Twenty-nine says: What are the diseases of the extraordinary channels like?

Answer: The *yang wei* links with the yang [channels], while the *yin wei* links with the yin [channels]. If yin and yang [*wei mai*] are not able to link themselves to their mutual [partners], one is upset and loses one's mind. One's [qi and blood flow will be] broad[34] and one will not be able to hold oneself up. If the *yang wei* is diseased, there is the bitterness of cold and heat. If the *yin wei* is diseased, there is the bitterness of heart pain. If the *yin qiao* is diseased, the yang [*qiao*] will be slack, while the yin [*qiao*] will be tense. If the *yang qiao* is diseased, the yin [*qiao*] will be slack and the yang [*qiao*] will be tense. If the *chong* is diseased, the qi will counterflow and in the interior there will be tension [or cramping]. If the conception [vessel] is diseased, internally there will be the bitterness of binding. Men will have the seven mountings, while

---

[34] In other words, one's qi and blood flow will be like a broad river which no longer flows with any power or force.

women will have conglomerations and gatherings. When the belt vessel is diseased, there is abdominal fullness, low back broadness [*i.e.*, lack of strength, and a feeling] as if sitting in water. This is what happens when the extraordinary channel eight vessels are diseased.

Thirty

Difficulty Thirty says: The constructive qi moves and, normally, does not the defensive qi follow it?

Answer: *The Classic* says humans receive their qi from grain. Grains enter the stomach and are then transmitted to the five viscera and six bowels. [Thus,] the five viscera and six bowels all receive their qi. The clear makes the constructive, while the turbid makes the defensive. The constructive moves within the vessels, while the defensive moves outside. The constructive moves in a circuit without [taking] a breath [*i.e.*, without ceasing]. Fifty [circuits] and [the constructive] returns to its great meeting [with the defensive]. Yin and yang mutually link, like a ring without an end. Thus it is understood that the constructive and defensive mutually follow one another.

Thirty-one

Difficulty Thirty-one says: The three burners, from where are they endowed and from where are they engendered? Where do they begin and where do they end? Where, in general, can they be treated? Can these be known?

Answer: The three burners are the passage-ways of water and grain, the end and beginning of [the circulation of] qi. The upper burner is located below the heart to below the diaphragm [ending] at the upper mouth of the stomach. It governs internalizing [*i.e.,* taking in] and does not exit [or discharge]. It is treated at Chest Center (*Dan Zhong,* CV 17), one inch and six *fen* below Jade Hall (*Yu Tang,* CV 18), straight in the fold between the two breasts. The middle burner is located [where] the stomach and middle venter are, not above and not below. It governs the rottening and ripening of water and grain. It is treated at the sides of the navel [*i.e., Tian Shu,* St 25]. The lower burner [begins] exactly at the upper mouth of the bladder. It rules the division and separation of clear and turbid. It governs exiting and does not internalize [*i.e.,* take in]. Thus it [serves as] a transmitting passageway. It is treated one inch below the navel. Therefore, this is what is called the three burners. They are the mansion in which are located the qi thoroughfares.

Thirty-two

Difficulty Thirty-two says: The five viscera are all of equal rank, yet only the heart and lungs are located above the diaphragm. Why is this?

Answer: The heart [is associated with] the blood, while the lungs [are associated with] the qi. The blood makes the constructive, while the qi makes the defensive. These mutually follow each other up and down and are called the constructive and defensive. These flow freely and move through the channels and network vessels and circulate through the external. Therefore, only the heart and lungs are located above the diaphragm.

Thirty-three

Difficulty Thirty-three says: The liver [is associated with] green and resembles wood. The lungs [are associated with] white and resemble metal. When the liver obtains water, it sinks. When wood obtains water, it floats. When the lungs obtain water, they float, while when metal obtains water, it sinks. What is the meaning of this?

Answer: The liver is not pure wood. *Yi jiao* [35] is the soft [*i.e.*, yin, partner] of *geng*. The large meaning [of *yi* and *geng*] is yin and yang, while the small meaning is husband and wife. [The liver] releases its faint yang and absorbs the faint yin qi, desiring the happiness of metal. It also moves mostly in the yin passageways. Therefore, when the liver obtains water it sinks.

The lungs are not pure metal. *Xin shang* is the soft [*i.e.*, yin, partner] of *bing*. The large meaning

---

[35] *Yi* is one of the 10 heavenly stems, while *jiao* is the musical note associated with wood. The 10 heavenly stems are divided into the five phases, with a yin and yang stem corresponding to each phase.

[of *xin* and *bing*] is yin and yang, while the small meaning is husband and wife. [The lungs] release their faint yin and, through marriage, approach fire, desiring the happiness of fire. They also move mostly through the yang passageways. Therefore, when the lungs obtain water, they float.

If the lungs mature, once again they sink, while if the liver matures, once again it floats. Why is this?

This is because we know that *xin* must return to *geng* and *yi* must return to *jia*.

Thirty-four

Difficulty Thirty-four says: The five viscera each have a sound, color, smell, and flavor. These can be known, can they not?

Answer: The *Shi Bian (The Ten Changes)*[36] says the liver's color is green, its smell is parched, its flavor is sour, its sound is shouting, and its fluid is tears. The heart's color is red, its smell is scorched, its flavor is bitter, its sound is speech, and its fluid is sweat. The spleen's color is yellow, its smell is aromatic, its flavor is sweet, its sound is singing, and its fluid is saliva. The lungs' color is white, their smell is putrid [or fishy], their flavor is acrid, their sound is crying, and their fluid is snivel. The kidneys' color is black, their smell is rotten, their flavor is salty, their sound is groaning, and their fluid is spittle. These are the five viscera sounds, colors, smells, and flavors.

The five viscera also have seven spirits. In which of them is each [of these spirits] stored?

---

[36] This is the name of an ancient medical book which is no longer existent.

Answer: The viscera store and are the abode of a person's spirit qi. The liver stores the *hun* [or ethereal soul]. The lungs store the *po* [or corporeal soul]. The heart stores the spirit. The spleen stores ideas and intelligence. And the kidneys store the essence and will.[37]

---

[37] I believe that "will" here should merely be understood as desire.

Thirty-five

Difficulty Thirty-five says: The five viscera each have a place, and the bowels all are mutually [situated] nearby. Only the heart and lungs are removed at a distance from the large intestine and small intestine. What does this mean?

Answer: *The Classic* says, heart, constructive; lungs, defensive. [Both the heart and lungs] connect with and move the yang qi. Therefore, they are lodged in the upper [burner]. The large intestine and small intestine conduct the yin qi and descend. Therefore, they are lodged in the lower [burner]. That is why [these paired viscera and bowels] are located so far away from each other.

Again, all the bowels are yang, [in theory,] places of clarity and cleanliness. However, the large intestine, small intestine, stomach, and urinary bladder all receive what is not clean. What is the meaning of this?

Answer: In terms of all the bowels, it is not said [they are places of clarity and cleanliness]. *The Classic* says the small intestine receives the exuberance [*i.e.,* surplus] of the bowels, while the large intestine transmits, drains, and moves [this surplus] through the passageways of the bowels. The gallbladder is the bowel of clarity and cleanliness. The stomach is the bowel of water and grains, and the urinary bladder is the bowel of fluids and humors. One bowel cannot have two designations. Therefore, one knows it is not [as stated in the question].

The small intestine is the bowel of the heart. The large intestine is the bowel of the lungs. The gallbladder is the bowel of the liver. The stomach is the bowel of the spleen. And the urinary bladder is the bowel of the kidneys. The small intestine is called the red intestine, while the large intestine is called the white intestine. The gallbladder is called the green intestine, the stomach is called the yellow intestine, and the urinary bladder is called the black intestine. These are under the command of the lower burner.[38]

---

[38] All the bowels are under the command of the lower burner qi since all their contents eventually enter the lower burner.

Thirty-six

Difficulty Thirty-six says: Each viscus has one ear [or entity]. Only the kidneys have two. Why is this?

Answer: The two kidneys are not both kidneys. The left one makes up the kidneys, while the right one makes up the lifegate. The lifegate is the abode of all the spirit essence. It is the place to which is tied the original qi. In males, it stores the essence. In females, it ties to the uterus. Hence know there is [really only] one kidney.

Thirty-seven

Difficulty Thirty-seven says: Where does the qi of the five viscera emit and arise and where does it flow to? This can be known can it not?

Answer: The five viscera are connected above with the nine orifices. Therefore, the lung qi flows freely to [or connects with] the nose. If the nose is harmonious, one can know aroma from fetor. The liver qi connects with the eyes. If the eyes are harmonious, one can know black from white. The spleen qi connects with the mouth. If the mouth is harmonious, one can know the flavor of grains. The heart qi connects with the tongue. If the tongue is harmonious, one can know the five flavors. The kidney qi connects with the ears. If the ears are harmonious, one can know the five notes.

If the five viscera are not harmonious, then they do not connect with the nine orifices. If the six bowels are not harmonious, retention and binding make welling abscesses. If evils are in the six bowels, the yang vessels are not harmonious. If the yang vessels are not harmonious, the qi is retained. If the qi is retained, the yang vessels become exuberant. If evils are in the five viscera, the yin vessels are not harmonious. If the yin vessels are not harmonious, the blood is retained. If the blood is retained, the yin vessels thus become exuberant.

If yin qi becomes greatly exuberant, yang qi will not obtain mutual construction.[39] Therefore, one speaks of checking. If the yang qi is greatly exuberant, the yin qi will not obtain mutual construction. Therefore, one speaks of bar. If yin and yang are both exuberant, neither will obtain construction from the other, and thus one speaks of bar and checking. If there is bar and checking, one will not obtain one's final destiny[40] but will die [prematurely].

---

[39] The word *ying*, here translated here as construction, also means to seek or run, as in running an office. Therefore, Unschuld translates this line as: "In case of a great surplus of influences in the yin [vessels], influences from the yang [vessels] cannot circulate [into the yin vessels]." In other words, this word *ying* may also be used to imply movement or circulation.

[40] Final destiny means one's heaven decreed span of life which should be around 100 years.

The Classic says the qi only moves through the five viscera and does not seek [or run] the six bowels. Why is that?

Answer: The movement of the qi is like the flow of water, never obtaining [*i.e.*, never coming to] a rest. Therefore, the yin vessels seek [or flow into] the five viscera, while the yang vessels seek the six bowels. This is like a ring without an end. Nobody knows its break. It ends and [yet] begins again. Hence there is no turning back and spilling over. A person's qi internally warms the viscera and bowels, while externally moistens the interstices.

Thirty-eight

Difficulty Thirty-eight says: There are five viscera but six bowels. Why is this?

Answer: Where it says there are six bowels, this is because of the triple burner. It is yet [another] divergence [or source] of original qi. It governs and grasps [*i.e.*, manages] all the qi. It has a name but no form. Its channel homes to the hand *shao yang*. It is the external bowel.[41] Hence it is said there are six bowels.

---

[41] External bowel means that it is the "bowel" on the external which contains all the other viscera and bowels.

Thirty-nine

Difficulty Thirty-nine says: *The Classic* says
there are five bowels and six viscera. Why is
this?

Answer: [Usually, one speaks of] six bowels,
but actually there are five bowels. [If one says
that] the five bowels also have six viscera, this
means the kidneys have two viscera. The left is
the kidney [*per se*], while the right is the lifegate.
The lifegate is called the abode of the essence
spirit. In males, it stores the essence, while in
females it ties to the uterus. Its qi and the
kidneys' communicate [or are common, *i.e.*, the
same]. Therefore, it is said there are six viscera.

[When it is said that] there are five bowels, what
does this mean?

Answer: The five viscera each have one bowel.
The triple burner is also a bowel. However, it

does not pertain to [one of] the five viscera. Therefore, it is said that there are five bowels.[42]

---

[42] In other words, when it is said there are six viscera, the kidney and lifegate are being counted as two separate but connected viscera. When it is said there are five bowels, the triple burner is not being included.

Forty

Difficulty Forty says: *The Classic* says the liver rules colors, the heart rules smells, the spleen rules flavors, the lungs rule sounds, and the kidneys rule fluids. The nose is the indicator of the lungs. [Yet] contrarily it knows aroma from fetor. The ears are the indicators of the kidneys, [yet] they hear sounds. What is the meaning of this?

Answer: The lungs are western direction metal. Metal is engendered by [the terrestrial branch] *si. Si* is southern direction fire. Fire is the heart, and the heart rules smell. Therefore, the nose knows aroma from fetor. The kidneys are northern direction water. Water is engendered by *shen. Shen* is western direction metal. Metal is the lungs. The lungs rule sound. Therefore, the ears hear sounds.

Forty-one

Difficulty Forty-one says: Only the liver has two lobes. To what does these correspond?

Answer: The liver is eastern direction wood. Wood is the spring. [During the spring,] the tens of thousands of things are born and come to life. [However,] they are still young and small. Their trace is not [yet] close to anything. [Spring] departs from *tai yin* [winter] but is still close [to it]. It is separated from *tai yang* [summer] but is not far [from it]. This is just like having two hearts, and, therefore, [the liver] has two lobes. This also corresponds to the leaves of trees [which are more than one].

Forty-two

Difficulty Forty-two says: What is the long and short [*i.e.*, length] of the intestines and stomach and which receives [*i.e.*, contains] more or less of water and grains?

Answer: The stomach is one cubit five inches large [*i.e.*, wide] and its diameter is five inches. Its length is two cubits and six inches. It is coiled horizontally and receives three *dou* and five *sheng* of water and grain. Within this, commonly it retains two *dou* of grain and one *dou* five *sheng* of water. The small intestine is two and a half inches large [or wide]. Its diameter is eight *fen* and [a little] less than half a *fen*. Its length is three *chang* and two cubits. It receives two *dou* and four *sheng* of grain and six *sheng* and three and [a little] more than half a *he* of water. The returning intestine is four inches large. Its diameter is one and a half inches. Its length is two *chang* and one cubit. It receives one *dou* of grain and seven and a half *sheng* of water. The broad intestine is eight inches large, and its diameter is two and a half inches. It is two cubits and eight inches long. It receives nine *sheng* and three and one eighth *he* of grain.

-84-

Therefore, the length of the intestines and stomach is five *chang*, eight cubits, and four inches. The combined grain and water received is eight *dou*, seven *sheng* and one eighth *he*. This is the long and short of the intestines and stomach and the numbers of water and grain they receive.

The liver weighs two *jin* and four *liang*. On the left it has three leaves [or lobes] and on the right four lobes, altogether seven lobes. It mainly stores the *hun* [or ethereal soul]. The heart weighs 12 *liang*. It has seven holes and three hairs within it. It is exuberant [*i.e.*, filled with] three *he* of essence juice. It mainly stores the spirit. The spleen weighs two *jin* and three *liang*. Its flat width is three inches. Its length is five inches. It has one half *jin* of scattered fat. It contains the blood, warms the five viscera, and mainly stores the mind. The lungs weigh three *jin* and three *liang*. They have six lobes and two ears or altogether eight lobes. They mainly store the *po* [or corporeal soul]. The kidneys have two entities. They weigh one *jin* and two *liang*. They mainly store the will. The gallbladder is located between the short lobes of the liver. It weighs three *liang* and three *chu*. It is exuberant [or filled with] three *he* of essence juice. The stomach weighs two *jin* and 14 *liang*. It curves, bending and extending. It is two cubits and six inches long, one cubit and five inches large, and its diameter is five inches. It is exuberant [or filled with] two *dou* of grain and one *dou* and five *sheng* of water. The small intestine weighs two *jin* and 14 *liang*. It is three *chang* and two cubits long, two and a half inches broad, and eight and [a little] less than half a *fen* in diameter. It lies folded, turning to the left with 16 bends. It is exuberant [or filled with] two *dou* and four *sheng* of grain and six *sheng* and three and more than a half *he* of water. The large intestine weighs three *jin* and 12 *liang*, is two *chang* and one cubit long, four inches broad, and one inch in diameter. It is located exactly at the navel, turning to the right with 16 bends. It is exuberant [or filled with] one *dou* of grain and seven and a half *sheng* of water. The urinary bladder weighs nine *liang* and two *chu*. Its longitudinal breadth is nine inches. It is exuberant [or filled with] nine *sheng* and nine *he* of urine. The mouth is two and a half inches broad. From the lips to the teeth is nine *fen* long.

From the teeth backward to the epiglottis is three and a half inches deep. [The oral cavity] holds, at most, five *he*. The tongue weighs 10 *liang*. It is seven inches long and two and a half inches broad. The throat gate [or esophagus] weighs 12 *liang*. It is two and a half inches broad. [From there] to the stomach is one cubit and six inches long. The windpipe weighs 12 *liang*, is two inches broad, and is one cubit and two inches long with nine joints. The anal gate weighs 12 *liang*, is eight *fen* large, and two and more than a half inches in diameter. It is two cubits and eight inches long. It receives nine *sheng* and three and one eighth *he* of grain.

Forty-three

Difficulty Forty-three says: If a person does not eat or drink for seven days, they die. Why is this?

Answer: A person's stomach retains two *dou* of grain and one *dou* and five *sheng* of water. Therefore, a level [*i.e.*, normal or healthy] person will go to the latrine two times per day and, in one [bowel] movement [evacuate] two and a half *sheng* or five *sheng* [total] in one day. In seven days, [they will evacuate] five [times] seven [or] three *dou* and five *sheng*. Thus their water and grains are finished. Hence, if a healthy person does not eat or drink for seven days and dies, their death is due to their water, grains, fluids, and humors all being finished [or used up].

Forty-four

Difficulty Forty-four says: Where are the seven thoroughfare[43] gates located?

Answer: The lips are the flying gate. The teeth are the door gate. The epiglottis is the inhalation gate. The stomach is the hastening gate. The lower mouth [or opening] of the great granary is the nether gate. The meeting of the large intestine and small intestine is the balustrade gate. The lower end [*i.e.*, the anus] is the *po* [or corporeal soul] gate. Therefore, there are seven thoroughfare gates.

---

[43] The word *chong* here also means an important place.

Forty-five

Difficulty Forty-five says: *The Classic* says [there are] eight meetings. What are they?

Answer: The bowels meet at Great Granary (*Tai Cang*, CV 12). The viscera meet at Free Rib (*Ji Xie*, Liv 13). The sinews meet at Yang Mound Spring (*Yang Ling Quan*, GB 34). The marrow meets at Severed Bone (*Jue Gu*, GB 39). The blood meets at Diaphragm Transport (*Ge Shu*, Bl 17). The bones meet at Great Shuttle (*Da Shu*, Bl 10). The vessels meet at Great Abyss (*Tai Yuan*, Lu 9). The qi meets at the triple burner externally, [at a point located at] one sinew[44] directly between the two breasts. If a heat disease is located internally, choose the qi hole of the meeting [point of the affected entity].

---

[44] Sinew here may mean a visible vein.

Forty-six

Difficulty Forty-six says: Old people lie down but do not sleep. Young, strong people sleep and do not wake. Why is this?

Answer: *The Classic* says the young and strong [have] exuberant blood and qi. Their muscles and flesh are glossy [or smooth], their qi passageways are freely flowing, and the movement of their constructive and defensive does not lose its constancy [or regularity]. Therefore, during the daytime they are sharp,[45] and at night, they do not wake. Old people's blood and qi are debilitated, their muscles and flesh are not glossy, and their passageways of constructive and defensive are choppy [or rough]. Therefore, during the day, they are not able to be sharp, while at night they do not sleep. Thus one [should] under-stand [why] the elderly cannot obtain sleep.

---

[45] The word sharp or clever, shrewd, proficient is *jing*, the same word for essence. Because young people have a lot of qi and blood, they also have a lot of essence.

Forty-seven

Difficulty Forty-seven says: Only peoples' faces are able to withstand cold. Why is this?

Answer: A person's head is the meeting of all yang. All the yin vessels arrive at the neck, chest, and center, and then return. Only all the yang vessels ascend to arrive at the head and ears. Hence the face can withstand cold.

Forty-eight

Difficulty Forty-eight says: People have three vacuities and three repletions. What does this mean?

Answer: One may have vacuity or repletion of the pulses, vacuity or repletion of diseases, or repletion or vacuity of examinations [*i.e.*, signs and symptoms. In terms of] vacuity and repletion of the pulses, soggy makes for vacuity, while tight and confined make for repletion. [In terms of] vacuity and repletion of diseases, exiting [of the righteous] makes for vacuity, while entry [of evils] makes for repletion. Speaking makes for vacuity, while not speaking [*i.e.*, taciturnity and withdrawal] make for repletion. Slackness makes for vacuity, while tension makes for repletion. [In terms of] the vacuity and repletion of examinations, sogginess [or softness] makes for vacuity and confinement [or hardness] makes for repletion. Itching makes for vacuity, while pain makes for repletion. External pain but internal pleasure [or comfort] makes for external repletion and internal vacuity. Internal pain and external pleasure make for internal repletion and external vacuity. Thus it is said of vacuity and repletion.

Forty-nine

Difficulty Forty-nine says: What is the difference between [when] the regular channels become diseased by themselves and [when] the five evils damage them?

Answer: *The Classic* says grief and anxiety, thinking and worry damage the heart. Bodily cold and chilled drinks damage the lungs. Angry qi counterflow and ascension without descension damage the liver. Eating and drinking and [over-]taxation and fatigue damage the spleen. Enduring sitting on damp earth or strong [exertion] and entering water damage the kidneys. This is [how] the regular channels may become diseased by themselves.

What is meant by the five evils?

Answer: To have been struck by wind, to have been damaged by summerheat, to have been [damaged by] eating and drinking and [over-]taxation and fatigue, to have been damaged by cold, to have been struck by dampness, these are called the five evils.

Take heart disease for example. How can one know this was obtained by being struck by the wind?

Answer: Their color [*i.e.*, facial complexion] must be red. Why do [I] say this? The liver rules the colors. Self-entry makes for green. [Evils] entering the heart makes for red. Entry of the lungs makes for white. Entry of the kidneys makes for black. If the liver makes for heart evils, therefore, one knows the color must be red. Their disease [also has] bodily heat and hypochondral fullness and pain. Their pulse is floating and bowstring.

How can one know [their disease] was obtained by being damaged by summerheat?

Answer: They must have a malign [or bad] odor. Why do [I] say this? The heart rules odors [or smells]. Self-entry makes for a scorched odor. [Evils] entering the spleen makes for an aromatic odor. Entry of the liver makes for a parched odor. Entry of the kidneys makes for a putrid odor. Entry of the lungs makes for a foul [or fishy] odor. Therefore, one knows that if the

heart is diseased by being damaged by
summerheat, [the patient] must have a malign
odor. Their disease [also has] bodily heat and
vexation and heart pain. Their pulse is floating,
large, and scattered.

How can one know [their disease] was obtained
by eating and drinking and [over-]taxation and
fatigue?

Answer: They must have a predilection for the
bitter flavor. Vacuity makes for no desire to eat.
Repletion makes for a desire to eat. Why do [I]
say this? The spleen rules flavors. [Evils]
entering the liver make for sour. Entry of the
heart makes for bitterness. Entry to the lungs
makes for acridity. Entry of the kidneys makes
for saltiness. Self-entry makes for sweet. Thus
one knows that spleen evils have entered the
heart and this makes for a predilection for the
bitter flavor. Their disease [also has] bodily heat
and bodily heaviness, a desire to lie down, and
non-contraction of the four limbs. Their pulse is
floating, large, and moderate [or relaxed].

How can one know [their disease] was obtained by damage due to cold?

Answer: They must talk nonsense and speak frenetically [*i.e.*, deliriously]. Why do [I] say this? The lungs govern sound. [Evils] entering the liver make for shouting. Entry of the heart makes for speaking. Entry of the spleen makes for singing. Entry of the kidneys makes for groaning. Self-entry makes for crying. Therefore, one knows lung evils have entered the heart, making for talking nonsense and speaking frenetically. Their disease [also has] bodily heat, sprinkling [*i.e.*, shivering], and aversion to cold. If severe, there is panting and coughing. Their pulse is floating, large, and choppy.

How can one know [their disease] was obtained by being struck by dampness?

Answer: They must have a predilection for sweating exiting which cannot be stopped. Why do [I] say this? The kidneys rule dampness. [Evils] entering the liver make for tears. Entry of the heart makes for sweat. Entry of the spleen makes for drool. Entry of the lungs makes for snivel. Self-entry makes for spittle. Thus, one knows kidney evils have entered the heart, making for sweating exiting which cannot be stopped. Their disease [also has] bodily heat, lower abdominal pain, foot and shin coldness and counterflow. Their pulse is sunken, soggy, and large.[46] This is the method of [knowing] the five evils.

---

[46] The soggy pulse is nowadays defined as a floating, fine, and forceless pulse. Therefore, to say that the pulse is sunken, large, meaning wide, and soggy in modern terms is a contradiction. Here, I believe soggy simply means relatively forceless.

Fifty

Difficulty Fifty says: Disease may have vacuity evils and they may have repletion evils. They may have thief evils, they may have faint [or slight] evils, and they may have regular evils. How are these distinguished?

Answer: [Those] coming from behind make for vacuity evils. [Those] coming from in front make for repletion evils. Those coming from where [or what] is not overcome make for thief evils. Those coming from what is overcome make for faint evils. And self-disease makes for regular evils. Why do [I] say so? Take, for example, heart disease. If obtained by wind stroke, this makes for vacuity evils. If obtained due to damage by summerheat, this makes for regular evils. If due to eating and drinking and [over-]taxation and fatigue, this makes for repletion evils. If obtained by damage due to cold, this makes for faint evils. If obtained by being struck by dampness, this makes for thief evils.

Fifty-one

Difficulty Fifty-one says: Diseases may have a desire for obtaining warmth or may have a desire for obtaining cold. There may be a desire for obtaining the sight of people or no desire for obtaining the sight of people. Each is not the same. How [can one know whether] the disease is located in the viscera or the bowels?

Answer: If the diseased desires to obtain cold and desires to see people, the disease is in the bowels. If the diseased desires to obtain warmth and does not desire to see people, the disease is in the viscera. What do [I] says this? The bowels are yang. Yang disease desires to obtain cold and also desires to see people. The viscera are yin. Yin disease desires to obtain warmth and also desires to have the doors shut and be alone. One is averse to hearing peoples' voices. Thus one can distinguish and know the diseases of the viscera and bowels.

Fifty-two

Difficulty Fifty-two says: When the viscera and the bowels emit disease [*i.e.*, become diseased], are they at root the same or different?

Answer: They are not the same.

Why aren't they the same?

Answer: Visceral diseases are stopped [*i.e.*, static] and are not variable. Such diseases do not depart from their place. Bowel diseases damage the Buddha[47] and rush around [making] sound. They ascend and descend, flow and move with no constancy to their abode. Therefore, from this one knows that the roots [of illnesses of] the viscera and bowels are not the same.

---

[47] According to Xu Da-chun, damaging the Buddha means they have no physical form.

Fifty-three

Difficulty Fifty-three says: *The Classic* says seven transmissions is death. Inter-transmission is life. What does this mean?

Answer: Seven transmissions [from viscus to viscus, mean] transmission to where [or what] they overcome [according to five phase theory]. Inter-transmission [means] transmitting to the child. Why do [I] say this? Take, for example, heart disease transmitted to the lungs. The lungs transmit to the liver [via the checking cycle]. The liver transmits to the spleen. The spleen transmits to the kidneys. The kidneys transmit to the heart. One viscus cannot be damaged twice. Therefore, it is said that seven transmissions is death. [If a disease] inter-transmits, it is transmitted to where [or what] it engenders. Take, for example, heart disease transmitted to the spleen. The spleen transmits to the lungs, the lungs transmit to the kidneys, the kidneys transmit to the liver, and the liver transmits to the heart. This is mutual transmission from mother to child. [The disease] circles and returns to its beginning like a ring with no end. Therefore, one says this is life.

Fifty-four

Difficulty Fifty-four says: Visceral diseases are difficult to treat, while bowel diseases are easy to treat. What is the meaning of this?

Answer: Visceral diseases are difficult to treat [because] they transmit to where [or what] they overcome. Bowel diseases are easy to treat [because] they transmit to their child. This is the same method [or principle] as the seven transmissions and inter-transmission [discussed above].

Fifty-five

Difficulty Fifty-five says: Diseases may have accumulations and they may have gatherings. How are these distinguished?

Answer: Accumulations [are] yin qi. Gatherings [are] yang qi. Therefore, yin sinks and is deep-lying [or hidden], while yang floats and stirs. The place where qi accumulates is called an accumulation. The place where qi gathers is called a gathering. Hence, accumulations are engendered in the five viscera, while gatherings are produced in the six bowels. Accumulations [are] yin qi. [Therefore,] they begin and stay constantly in the place they were emitted. Their pain does not separate [or leave] its location. Their upper and lower [borders] have [palpable] ending and beginning places, while their left and right [sides] have [definite] limits. Gatherings [are] yang qi. They develop without roots. Their upper and lower [borders] are without stay or stop, and their pain is not constant [or fixed] in location. Thus can one distinguish and know accumulations and gatherings.

Fifty-six

Difficulty Fifty-six says: Does each of the accumulations of the five viscera have its own name? In what month and on what day are they obtained [or contracted]?

Answer: The accumulation of the liver is called fat qi. It is located in the left hypochondrium. It is like an overturned cup. It has a head and foot. If it endures [a long time] without healing, the person emits [or develops] cough counterflow, tetany, and malaria-like [symptoms]. Continuing a year, they do not end. They are obtained in late summer on *wu* and *ji* days. Why do [I] say so? Lung disease transmits to the liver. The liver must transmit this to the spleen. The spleen is the right proper king of late summer, and the king does not receive [or accept] evils. [Therefore,] the liver desires to once again recycle [the disease] to the lungs, but the lungs are unwilling to accept [them]. Thus they are retained and bind, making an accumulation, and hence we can know that fat qi is obtained on *wu* and *ji* days in late summer.

The accumulation of the heart is called deep-lying beam. It arises above the navel. It is as large as the forearm. It ascends to arrive below the heart. If it endures [a long time] without healing, the person [has] heart vexation. It is obtained in the fall on *geng* and *xin* days. Why do [I] say this? Kidney disease is transmitted to the heart. The heart must transmit this to the lungs. The lungs are the right proper king of fall, and the king does not receive evils. [Therefore,] the heart desires to recycle [these evils] to the kidneys again, but the kidneys are unwilling to accept them. Hence, they are retained and bind, making an accumulation. Thus we can know that deep-lying beams are obtained on *geng* and *xin* days in the fall.

The accumulation of the spleen is called glomus qi. It is located in the stomach duct and is several times larger than a bowl. If it endures [a long time] without healing, the per-son has inability to contract the four limbs and the emission of yellow jaundice. Eating and drinking do not make the muscles and skin. This is obtained in winter on *ren* and *gui* days. Why do [I] say this? Liver disease is transmitted to the spleen. The spleen must transmit this to the kidneys. The kidneys are the right proper king of winter, and the king does not accept evils. [Therefore,] the spleen desires to recycle [these evils] to the liver again, but the liver is unwilling to accept them. Thus they are retained and bind, making an accumulation. Hence we can know that glomus qi is obtained in the winter on *ren* and *gui* days.

The accumulation of the lungs is called rushing respiration. It is located in the right hypochondrium. It is several times larger than a cup. If it endures [a long time] without healing, the person shivers with [alternating] cold and heat, has panting and coughing, and lung congestion.[48] This is obtained in spring on *jia* and *yi* days. Why do [I] say this? Heart disease is transmitted to the lungs. The lungs must transmit [this] to the liver. The liver is the right proper king of spring, and the king does not accept evils. [Therefore,] the lungs desire to recycle [these evils] to the heart again, but the

---

[48] The *Jia Yi Jing* (*Systematic Classic*) and the *Mai Jing* (*Pulse Classic*) both say lung welling abscess.

heart is unwilling to receive them. Thus they are retained and bind, making an accumulation. Therefore, we can know that rushing respiration is obtained in spring on *jia* and *yi* days.

The accumulation of the kidneys is called running piglet. It is emitted in the lower abdomen and ascends to arrive below the heart. It is like a piglet in shape. Possibly [*i.e.,* sometimes] it ascends and possibly it descends at no [definite] times. If it endures [for a long time] without ending, the person has panting counterflow, bone wilting, and scanty qi. This is obtained in the summer on *bing* and *ding* days. Why do [I] say this? Spleen disease is transmitted to the kidneys. The kidneys must transmit [this] to the heart. The heart is the suitable king of summer, and the king does not accept evils. [Therefore,] the kidneys desire to recycle [these evils] to the spleen again, but the spleen is unwilling to accept them. Hence, they are retained and bind, making an accumulation. Thus we can know that running piglet is obtained in the summer on *bing* and *ding* days.

Fifty-seven

Difficulty Fifty-seven says: How many kinds of discharge [or diarrhea] are there? They each have a name, do they not?

Answer: There are five kinds of discharge [or diarrhea] and their names are not the same. There is stomach discharge, spleen discharge, large intestine discharge, small intestine discharge, and large conglomeration discharge. [There is also something] called after heaviness [or tenesmus. In] stomach discharge, food and drink are not transformed and the color [of the stools] is yellow. In spleen diarrhea, there is abdominal distention and fullness, the discharge pours [like water], and eating results in vomiting and spitting counterflow. In large intestine discharge, after eating, there is a hard-pressed [feeling or cramps] and the stools are colored white. There is borborygmus and cutting pain. In small intestine discharge, there is pus and blood [when] urinating and defecating and lower abdominal pain. In large conglomeration discharge, there is interior tension [or cramping] and tenesmus. Numerous [times] one arrives at the latrine but is not able

to defecate. Within the stalk [or penis] there is
pain. This is the essential method of the five
discharges [or types of diarrhea].

Fifty-eight

Difficulty Fifty-eight says: How many kinds of damage due to cold are there, and are the pulses changed [by these or] not?

Answer: There are five damages due to cold. They are wind stroke, damage by cold, damp warmth, heat disease, and warm disease, and the bitterness [*i.e.*, suffering] in each is not the same. [As for] the wind stroke pulses, in the yang [position], it is floating and slippery. In the yin, it is soggy and weak. [In terms of] the pulses of damp warmth, in the yang, it is soggy and weak. In the yin, it is small and tense. [In terms of] the pulses of damage by cold, in the yin and yang both are exuberant, tight, and choppy [or rough. As for] the pulses of heat disease, both yin and yang are floating. In the floating [level, the pulse is] slippery. Deep, it is scattered and choppy. [In terms of] the pulses of warm disease, [this kind of disease] moves through all the channels. [Therefore,] one cannot know which channel a stirring belongs to. In that case, follow the channel(s) where [the evils] are located and choose [those channels].

When damage due to cold has sweat exit, it is cured. Precipitate and there will be death. [In cases where] sweat exiting [would lead to] death, precipitating cures. Why is this?

Answer: If yang is vacuous and yin is exuberant, sweat exiting cures but precipitating results in death. [In cases where] yang is exuberant and yin is vacuous, exiting of sweat [causes] death, but precipitating cures.

What are the indicators of cold and heat disease?

Answer: If there is skin cold and heat, the skin cannot approach the mat, the hair is scorched, and the nose is dry, do not obtain sweating. If there is muscle cold and heat, the skin is painful and the lips and tongue are dry. No sweating. If there is bone cold and heat, the disease is not quiet [*i.e.,* does not rest] anywhere. Sweat pours ceaselessly and the roots of the teeth are dry and painful.

Fifty-nine

Difficulty Fifty-nine says: How are mania and epilepsy distinguished?

Answer: At the beginning emission [or outbreak] of mania, there is little lying down and no hunger. One [speaks of] oneself [as if] elevated and worthy [of honor]. One discriminates [or points out] one's [special] intelligence and one behaves in an arrogant and haughty way. One frenetically smiles, sings, and is happy and frenetically moves about without a break. During the initial outbreak of epilepsy, the mind is not happy. One lies stiffly, staring straight [ahead]. The pulses of the three positions yin and yang are all exuberant.

Sixty

Difficulty Sixty says: [Among] the diseases of the head and heart, there are inversion pain and true pain. What does this mean?

Answer: If the hand three yang vessels receive [*i.e.*, contract] wind cold and this lies deeply, is retained, and is not removed, this may lead to what is called reversal headache. [If these evils] enter and continue to the brain, this is called true headache. If the qi of [any of] the five viscera mutually turn against [the heart], that is called reversal heart pain. If the pain is severe but located [only] in the heart and the hands and feet are green-blue, this is called true heart pain. If true heart pain emits [or occurs] at dawn, death is at sunset. If it occurs at sunset, death is at dawn [the next morning].

Sixty-one

Difficulty Sixty-one says: *The Classic* says looking and knowing [the patient's diagnosis] is called spirit[-like or godly]. Hearing and knowing is called sage[-like]. Questioning and knowing is called workman[-like]. Palpating the pulses and knowing is called clever. What does this mean?

Answer: Those who look and know look at the appearance of the five colors in order to know [the person's] disease. Those who hear and know hear the five notes in order to distinguish their disease. Those who question and know question [the person's] desire for the five flavors in order to know where the disease has arisen and where it is located. Those who palpate the pulse and know examine the inch mouth to see their vacuity and repletion and hence know in what viscus or bowel their disease is located. When *The Classic* says those knowing from external [manifestations] are called sage[-like], while those knowing from internal [manifestations] are called spirit[-like], this is what it means.

Sixty-two

Difficulty Sixty-two says: The visceral
[channels of] wells and brooks [etc.] have five,
while only the bowels have six. What does this
mean?

Answer: The bowels [are] yang. The three
burners move through all the yang. Therefore,
there is an additional one transport [point on
the yang channels] called the origin [or source.
When it is said] the bowels have six, this is
because the three burners have one qi in
common in addition [to those of the other five].

Sixty-three

Difficulty Sixty-three says: The *Shi Bian (The Ten Changes)* says the five viscera and six bowels' [points from] brook [to] uniting all begin with the well. Why is this?

Answer: The wells [correspond to] the eastern direction and spring, the beginning of life of the tens of thousands of things when all the *qi* [insects] move, panting and breathing, the *quan* [insects] fly, and the *juan* [insects] stir. All things that come to life, do not come to life other than in the spring. Therefore, numbering the [dates of the] year begins in the spring and numbering the days begins with *jia*. Therefore, the wells make for the beginnings [of all the channels of the five viscera and six bowels].

Sixty-four

Difficulty Sixty-four says: The *Shi Bian (The Ten Changes)* also says yin wells are wood, while yang wells are metal. Yin brooks are fire, while yang brooks are water. Yin streams are earth, while yang streams are wood. Yin rivers are metal, while yang rivers are fire. And yin uniting [points] are water, while yang uniting [points] are earth. Thus yin and yang are all not the same. What is the meaning of this?

Answer: This is a matter of hardness and softness. Yin wells are *yi* wood, while yang wells are *geng* metal. The yang wells' *geng* is the *geng* of the hardness of *yi*. The yin wells' *yi* is the *yi* of the softness of *geng*. *Yi* makes for wood. Therefore, one speaks of the yin wells as wood. *Geng* makes for metal. Therefore, one speaks of the yang wells as metal. The same applies to all the rest.

Sixty-five

Difficulty Sixty-five says: *The Classic* says the place of exiting makes for the wells. The place of entering makes for the uniting. What kind of method [or principle] is this?

Answer: The place of exiting makes for the well. The well [corresponds to] the eastern direction and spring, the beginning of life of the tens of thousands of things. Therefore, it is said that the place of exiting makes for the well. The place of entry makes for the uniting. The uniting [corresponds to] the northern direction and winter, when yang qi enters and is stored. Therefore, it is said that the place of entering makes for the uniting.

Sixty-six

Difficulty Sixty-six says: *The Classic* says the lungs's origin exits from Great Abyss (*Tai Yuan*, Lu 9). The heart's origin exits from Great Mound (*Da Ling*, Per 7). The liver's origin exits from Supreme Surge (*Tai Chong*, Liv 3). The spleen's origin exits from Supreme White (*Tai Bai*, Sp 3). The kidneys' origin exits from Great Ravine (*Tai Xi*, Ki 3). The *shao yin*'s origin exits from Protuberant Bone (*Dui Gu*, Ht 7). The gallbladder's origin exits from Hill Ruins (*Qiu Xu*, GB 40). The stomach's origin exits from Surging Yang (*Chong Yang*, St 42). The triple burner's origin exits from Yang Pool (*Yang Chi*, TB 4). The urinary bladder's origin exits from Capital Bone (*Jing Gu*, Bl 64). The large intestine's origin exits from Union Valley (*He Gu*, LI 4). The small intestine's origin exits from Wrist Bone (*Wan Gu*, SI 4).

On all 12 channels, the stream [points] make for the origins. Why?

Answer: All the five viscera stream [points] are the triple burner's place of movement where the qi is retained and stops.

Why do the stream [points] of the triple burner's place of movement [also] make for the origin [points]?

Answer: Below the navel is the moving qi between the kidneys, a person's life destiny and the root of the 12 channels. Therefore, it is called the origin. The triple burner is the special messenger of this original qi, governing the free flow and movement of the three qi through the five viscera and six bowels. Origin is an honorific designation of the triple burner. Hence, the place where [its qi stops and halts makes for the origin. [Whenever] the five viscera and six bowels have a disease, one should always choose their origin [points].

Sixty-seven

Difficulty Sixty-seven says: The *mu* [points] of the five viscera are all located on the yin [side of the body], while their transport [points] are located on the yang. What is the meaning of this?

Answer: Yin disease moves [to] the yang, while yang disease moves [to] the yin. Therefore, the *mu* are located on the yin, while the transports are located on the yang.

Sixty-eight

Difficulty Sixty-eight says: The five viscera and six bowels all have wells, brooks, streams, rivers, and uniting [points]. What [illnesses] do these places all govern?

Answer: *The Classic* says the place of exiting makes for the wells, the place of flowing makes for the brooks, the place of pouring makes for the streams, the place of movement makes for the rivers, and the place of entering makes for the uniting [points]. The wells rule fullness below the heart. The brooks rule bodily heat. The streams rule bodily heaviness and joint pain. The rivers rule panting and coughing, cold and heat. And the uniting [points] rule counterflow qi and discharge [or diarrhea]. These are the five viscera and six bowels' wells, brooks, streams, river, and uniting [points] places and the diseases they govern.

Sixty-nine

Difficulty Sixty-nine says: *The Classic* says for vacuity, supplement. For repletion, drain. If there is no repletion and no vacuity, choose the channel. What does this mean?

Answer: For vacuity, supplement the mother. For repletion, drain the child. First, supplement, and afterwards drain. If there is no vacuity and no repletion, [this means that] a regular channel has engendered disease by itself and has not been struck by evils. [Thus,] one should choose its own channel. Therefore, *The Classic* says choose the channel.

Seventy

Difficulty Seventy says: In spring and summer, prick shallowly; in fall and winter, prick deeply. What does this mean?

Answer: In the spring and summer, the yang qi is located above and humans' qi is also located above. Therefore, one should shallowly aim. In the fall and winter, the yang qi is located below and humans' qi is also located below. Therefore, one should deeply aim.

In spring and summer it is well-known [one should] deliver one [or some] yin, while in fall and winter, it is well-known [one should] deliver one [or some] yang. What does this mean?

Answer: Spring and summer are warm [and, therefore] one must deliver one yin. [To do this,] initially descend the needle, deeper [and deeper] until arriving at the region of the kidneys and liver, obtain the qi, and lead and hold the yin [to the yang]. The fall and winter are cold [and, therefore] one must deliver one yang. [To do this,] initially insert the needle shallowly and floating till arriving at the region of the heart and lungs. Obtain the qi and push the yang internally [to the yin]. This is what is spoken of as having to deliver one yin in spring and summer and having to deliver one yang in winter and fall.

Seventy-one

Difficulty Seventy-one says: *The Classic* says [when] pricking the constructive, do not damage the defensive. [When] pricking the defensive, do not damage the constructive. What does this mean?

Answer: [When] needling yang [*i.e.*, the defensive], prick with the needle lying down. [When] pricking yin [*i.e.*, the constructive], first use the left hand to gather and press the location of the transport [point] where the constructive is to be needled. [As soon as] the qi is scattered, insert the needle. This makes for pricking the constructive without damaging the defensive and pricking the defensive without damaging the constructive.

Seventy-two

Difficulty Seventy-two says: *The Classic* says if one can know if the qi meets or follows, one can regulate it. The formula [or method] of regulating the qi must be located in yin and yang. What does this mean?

Answer: When speaking of meeting and following, one [must] understand the flow and movement of the constructive and defensive and of the going and coming of the channels and vessels. Following [*i.e.,* based on their] counterflow and proper flow, one acts. Therefore, it is called meeting and following. [The statement that] the method of regulating the qi must exist in yin and yang [means that] one must understand whether [the disease] is internal or external, exterior or interior, regulating it following its yin or yang. Therefore, it is said that the method of regulating the qi must exist in yin and yang.

Seventy-three

Difficulty Seventy-three says: All the well [points are located where] the muscles and flesh are shallow and thin and [where] the qi is scanty and, [therefore,] insufficient to do [anything]. So how to prick [them]?

Answer: All the well [points] are wood, and all the brooks are fire. Fire is the child of wood. [Thus, if one] must prick the wells, do this by draining the brooks. Therefore, *The Classic* says, those that are supplemented, it is not OK to drain. Those that are drained, it is not OK to supplement. That is what is meant here.

Seventy-four

Difficulty Seventy-four says: *The Classic* says in spring prick the wells, in summer prick the brooks, in late summer prick the streams, in fall prick the rivers, and in winter prick the uniting [points]. What does this mean?

Answer: In spring, prick the wells [if] evils are located in the liver. In summer, prick the brooks [if] evils are located in the heart. In late summer, prick the streams [if] evils are located in the spleen. In fall, prick the rivers [if] evils are located in the lungs. In winter, prick the uniting [points if] evils are located in the kidneys.

Why are the liver, heart, spleen, lungs, and kidneys each tied to the spring, summer, fall, and winter [respectively]?

Answer: One disease in [any of] the five viscera may often have five [indicators]. Take, for example, liver disease. A green color [indicates] the liver. A parched odor [indicates] the liver. A predilection for sour [indicates] the liver. A predilection for shouting [indicates] the liver. And a tendency to tears [indicates] the liver.

Since there are so many diseases, one cannot exhaustively speak [of each. However,] the four times [or seasons] have numbers [*i.e.*, definite correspondences] and [all these illnesses] are also tied to spring, summer, fall, and winter [and thus to their corresponding phases, viscera, and points on the channels]. The important subtleties of needling are located in [*i.e.*, are as fine as] autumn hairs [or down].

Seventy-five

Difficulty Seventy-five says: *The Classic* says
that, if the eastern direction is replete and the
western direction is vacuous, drain the south
and supplement the north. What does this
mean?

Answer: Metal, wood, water, fire, and earth
should [all] mutually level [or normalize one
another]. The eastern direction [corresponds to]
wood, while the western direction [corresponds
to] metal. When wood is on the point of
repletion, metal should level it. When fire is on
the point of repletion, water should level it. If
earth is on the point of repletion, wood should
level it. If metal is on the point of repletion, fire
should level it. And if water is on the point of
repletion, earth should level it. The eastern
direction [corresponds to] wood. Therefore, one
knows the liver is replete [if wood is replete].
The western direction [corresponds to] metal.
Therefore, one knows the lungs are vacuous [if
metal is vacuous]. [In that case,] drain southern
fire and supplement northern water. Southern
fire is fire, the child of wood. Northern water is
water, the mother of wood. Water overcomes

fire, and the child is able [to make] the mother replete, while the mother is able [to make] the child vacuous. Therefore, drain fire and supplement water if one desires to obtain metal's leveling of wood. *The Classic* says [that if one is] not able to treat vacuity, what question is there [of treating all] the rest [of diseases]? This is what this means.

Seventy-six

Difficulty Seventy-six says: What is the meaning of supplementing and discharging? When one must supplement, from whence should one get the qi? When one must drain, where should one put [or take] the qi?

Answer: When one must supplement, get the qi from the defensive. When one must drain, take the qi from the constructive. If yang qi is insufficient and yin qi has a surplus, first one should supplement the yang and afterwards drain the yin. If yin qi is insufficient and yang qi has a surplus, first one should supplement the yin and afterwards drain the yang. That the constructive and defensive should connect and move free-flowingly is what's essential.

Seventy-seven

Difficulty Seventy-seven says: *The Classic* says the superior worker treats [what's] not diseased. The mediocre worker treats [what's] already diseased. What does this mean?

Answer: Where it is said treat [what's] not diseased, [this means that when] one sees a disease of the liver, one should know that the liver must transmit [this disease] to the spleen. Therefore, one should first replete the spleen qi before [the spleen] obtains and receives evils from the liver. This is what's called treating [what's] not diseased. When a mediocre worker sees a disease of the liver, not knowing about mutual transmission, [they will, with] one heart [*i.e.*, single-mindedly], treat the liver. This is what's called treating [what's] already diseased.

Seventy-eight

Difficulty Seventy-eight says: Needling has supplementation and drainage. What does this mean?

Answer: Supplementing and draining methods do not require exhaling and inhaling [when] exiting and inserting the needles. [Those who] know how to do needling speak of the left. [Those who] do not know how to do needling speak of the right. When pricking, one should first use the left hand to press the location of the constructive transport [point] to be needled. Sending forth and exerting [pressure], descend the fingernail. [When] the qi comes, its form is like stirring vessels [*i.e.*, a pulse. Then can one] propitiously prick with the needle. [After] obtaining the qi, push [it] internally. This is called supplementation. Stirring [*i.e.*, moving the needle] and then withdrawing it is called drainage. If the qi is not obtained, therefore [seek it] in males externally and in females internally. If one [still] does not obtain the qi, this makes for 10 [out of 10] dying and being untreatable.

Seventy-nine

Difficulty Seventy-nine says: [When] *The Classic* says meeting and wresting, how can one [rest] quiet that one has obtained no [*i.e.*, not caused] vacuity? [When] following and aiding, how can one [rest] quiet that one has obtained no repletion? Vacuity [compared to] repletion is like obtaining [compared to] losing. Repletion [compared to] vacuity is like having to not [having]. What does this mean?

Answer: To meet and wrest, drain the child. To follow and aid, supplement the mother. Take, for example, heart disease. Draining the hand heart governor stream [point] is called meeting and wresting. Supplementing the hand heart governor well [point] is called following and aiding. Where repletion and vacuity are spoken of, the meaning is hard and soggy [or soft]. If the qi comes replete and hard [or firm], this is [like] obtaining [or gaining. If it comes] soggy and vacuous, this is [like] losing. Therefore, it is said like obtaining and like losing.

Eighty

Difficulty Eighty says: *The Classic* says [when it] is apparent, insert; [when] apparent, exit. What does this mean?

Answer: Where it is said [when] apparent, insert, it means [when] the coming and arrival of the qi is apparent to the left hand, then insert the needle. [After] the needle has been inserted and it is apparent that the qi is finished [or departed], then exit the needle. This is what is meant by [when] it is apparent, insert, and [when] it is apparent, exit.

Eighty-one

Difficulty Eighty-one says: *The Classic* says do not replete repletion [or make more] vacuous vacuity, [thus causing] detriment [to what is] insufficient and boosting [that which has] a surplus. Does this [concern] the inch mouth pulses? Or [does it refer to] self[-made] diseases having [*i.e.*, those resulting from incorrect treatment of] vacuity and repletion? [Further,] what do detriment and boosting mean?

Answer: This [statement] is [or refers to] diseases. It does not mean the inch mouth pulses. It means self[-made] diseases having vacuity and repletion. Take, for example, liver repletion and lung vacuity. The liver [corresponds to] wood, while the lungs [correspond to] metal. Metal and wood should make each other mutually level, and one [should] know how [to make] metal level wood. Take, as [another] example, lung repletion and liver vacuity with faint and scanty qi. If one uses needles not to supplement the liver but contrarily [to make even] heavier the repletion of the lungs, this is [what is] spoken of as repleting repletion [and making more] vacuous vacuity, [causing] detriment [to what is] insufficient and boosting [that which] has a surplus. This is the harm of [or caused by] mediocre workers.

CURING DEPRESSION NATURALLY
WITH CHINESE MEDICINE
by Rosa Schnyer & Bob Flaws
ISBN 0-936185-94-5

CURING FIBROMYALGIA
NATURALLY WITH CHINESE
MEDICINE
by Bob Flaws
ISBN 1-891845-09-8

CURING HAY FEVER NATURALLY
WITH CHINESE MEDICINE
by Bob Flaws
ISBN 0-936185-91-0

CURING HAY FEVER NATURALLY
WITH CHINESE MEDICINE
by Bob Flaws
ISBN 0-936185-91-0

CURING HEADACHES NATURALLY
WITH CHINESE MEDICINE
by Bob Flaws
ISBN 0-936185-95-3

CURING IBS NATURALLY WITH
CHINESE MEDICINE
by Jane Bean Oberski
ISBN 1-891845-11-X

CURING INSOMNIA NATURALLY
WITH CHINESE MEDICINE
by Bob Flaws
ISBN 0-936185-86-4

CURING PMS NATURALLY
WITH CHINESE MEDICINE
by Bob Flaws
ISBN 0-936185-85-6

THE DIVINE FARMER'S MATERIA
MEDICA:
A Translation of the Shen Nong Ben Cao
translation by Yang Shou-zhong
ISBN 0-936185-96-1

THE DIVINELY RESPONDING
CLASSIC:
A Translation of the Shen Ying Jing from
Zhen Jiu Da Cheng
trans. by Yang Shou-zhong & Liu Feng-ting
ISBN 0-936185-55-4

DUI YAO: THE ART OF COMBINING
CHINESE HERBAL MEDICINALS
by Philippe Sionneau
ISBN 0-936185-81-3

ENDOMETRIOSIS, INFERTILITY AN
TRADITIONAL CHINESE MEDICIN
A Laywoman's Guide
by Bob Flaws
ISBN 0-936185-14-7

THE ESSENCE OF LIU FENG-WU'S
GYNECOLOGY
by Liu Feng-wu, translated by Yang Shou
zhong
ISBN 0-936185-88-0

EXTRA TREATISES BASED ON
INVESTIGATION & INQUIRY:
A Translation of Zhu Dan-xi's Ge Zhi
Lun
translation by Yang Shou-zhong
ISBN 0-936185-53-8

FIRE IN THE VALLEY: TCM Diagnos
& Treatment of Vaginal Diseases
by Bob Flaws
ISBN 0-936185-25-2

FU QING-ZHU'S GYNECOLOGY
trans. by Yang Shou-zhong and Liu Da-w
ISBN 0-936185-35-X

FULFILLING THE ESSENCE:
A Handbook of Traditional &
Contemporary Treatments for Female
Infertility
by Bob Flaws
ISBN 0-936185-48-1

GOLDEN NEEDLE WANG LE-TIN(
A 20th Century Master's Approach t
Acupuncture
by Yu Hui-chan and Han Fu-ru, trans. b
Shuai Xue-zhong
ISBN 0-936185-789-3

A GUIDE TO GYNECOLOGY
by Ye Heng-yin, trans. by Bob Flaws and
Shuai Xue-zhong
ISBN 1-891845-19-5

160 ESSENTIAL CHINESE HERBAL
PATENT MEDICINES
by Bob Flaws
ISBN 1-891945-12-8

230 ESSENTIAL CHINESE
MEDICINALS
by Bob Flaws
ISBN 1-891845-03-9

630 QUESTIONS & ANSWERS
ABOUT CHINESE HERBAL
MEDICINE:
A Workbook & Study Guide
by Bob Flaws
ISBN 1-891845-04-7

750 QUESTIONS & ANSWERS
ABOUT ACUPUNCTURE
Exam Preparation & Study Guide
by Fred Jennes
ISBN 1-891845-22-5